2003

RESEARCH IN
HEALTH CARE

RESEARCH IN HEALTH CARE

Design, Conduct and Interpretation
of Health Services Research

I.K. Crombie
with
H.T.O. Davies

Department of Epidemiology & Public Health,
Ninewells Hospital & Medical School,
University of Dundee, UK

JOHN WILEY & SONS

Chichester • New York • Brisbane • Toronto • Singapore

Other Wiley Editorial Offices

John Wiley & Sons, Inc., 605 Third Avenue,
New York, NY 10158-0012, USA

Jacaranda Wiley Ltd, 33 Park Road, Milton,
Queensland 4064, Australia

John Wiley & Sons (Canada) Ltd, 22 Worcester Road,
Rexdale, Ontario M9W 1L1, Canada

John Wiley & Sons (Asia) Pte Ltd, 2 Clementi Loop #02-01,
Jin Xing Distripark, Singapore 0512

Library of Congress Cataloging-in-Publication Data

Crombie, I.K.
    Research in health care : a practical approach to the design,
conduct, and interpretation of health services research / I.K.
Crombie with H.T.O. Davies; foreword by Michael Peckham.
        p.   cm.
    Includes bibliographical references and index.
    ISBN 0-471-96259-7 (pbk. : alk. paper)
    1. Medical care — Research — Methodology. I. Davies, H.T.O.
II. Title.
    [DNLM: 1. Health Services Reseach–methods. 2. Research Design.
3. Communication. W 84.3 C945r 1996]
    RA440.85.C76   1996
    362.1'072–dc20
    DNLM/DLC
    for Library of Congress   95-42359
                                                                    CIP

British Library Cataloguing in Publication Data
A catalogue record for this book is available from the British Library

ISBN 0-471-96259-7
Typeset in 10/12pt Palatino by Mayhew Typesetting, Rhayader, Powys
Printed and bound in Great Britain by Biddles Ltd, Guildford and King's Lynn
This book is printed on acid-free paper responsibly manufactured from sustainable
forestation, for which at least two trees are planted for each one used for paper production.

CONTENTS

FOREWORD

The role of research and development in shaping health services as they seek to adapt to major change is now receiving the recognition it deserves. With this recognition, however, comes the challenge of ensuring that the outputs of R&D demonstrably influence policy, clinical practice and management. The success of health services research therefore depends upon the precision with which problems appropriate for research are identified, the rigour with which they are tackled and the mechanisms in place to secure practical use of the results.

The analysis of health service issues that might be resolved by research and the application of appropriate investigative methods are intellectually challenging and should be seen as a partner to cell, molecular and clinical science, and other areas of research relevant to health. Arbitrary distinctions between basic and applied health research obscure a balanced view of the scientific basis of health and health care. Indeed, a fundamental weakness of the past has been the failure to make appropriate use of scientific methods to ensure that the products of science and technology are fully exploited in practice.

As the recent House of Lords report, 'Medical Research and the NHS Reforms', has observed: *'Our evidence leads us to conclude that this is an exciting time to be a researcher working in or with the NHS . . . health services research is . . . making great strides'*. Broadening the scope of research to encompass issues, for example relating to the organisation and management of services or to the deployment of staff, requires an understanding of the strengths, weaknesses and appropriate use of the available repertoire of research methods. It is in this context that *Research in Health Care* is a most welcome contribution. It is also timely given the high level of current interest in evidence-based health care and in the training and careers of researchers in the previously neglected field of health services research.

Professor Sir Michael Peckham
Director of Research and Development,
Department of Health

PREFACE

Health services research was, until recently, a discipline which was largely ignored. But a series of events and initiatives within the NHS over the last decade have placed it high on the agenda. The future will see a mushrooming of activity in health services research, in which all health care professionals will be encouraged to participate. This book provides a practical guide to the design, conduct and interpretation of research into the delivery of health care. It tackles the *what, why* and *how* of research: what to do to conduct successful research; why it needs to be carried out in a particular way; and how this can be achieved.

The book presents an overview of health services research, to clarify its nature and the range of problems it investigates. The characteristics of high quality research are also addressed, particularly the central position of a good research question. Next the several methods available for health research are described. Advice is given on how to employ these methods, where the pitfalls lie and how they can be avoided. The practical issues involved in collecting data and conducting research studies are reviewed separately. In the final chapters, strategies are presented for the analysis, interpretation and publication of study findings.

Textbooks on research are often intimidating, proceeding from definitions of technical terms to formal expositions on the methods of research. This book is different. It avoids technical terms wherever possible, explaining the ideas underlying these terms in plain English. Examples of published studies are used extensively to illustrate the ideas presented, placing research firmly in the context of health care delivery. The book is fully referenced, and the reader is guided to relevant literature from a range of related fields.

The book provides a step-by-step guide for those who wish to conduct research or interpret published studies. It is intended for all health care professionals, including doctors, nurses, and the professions allied to medicine.

ACKNOWLEDGEMENTS

This book has its origins in a conversation with a colleague, Fiona Williams, on the research needs of health care professionals. Fiona, along with Charles Florey, Sarah Cunningham-Burley and Linda Irving, gave many helpful comments on the text. Johanne Phillips provided invaluable assistance with the references. Any book on research builds on the ideas and observations of many generations of scientists and health professionals. This book has benefited greatly from many published works, particularly those by PB Medawar and J Calnan. Much of the reading for this book was carried out while the author was on sabbatical in New Zealand, and he is grateful to the members of the Department of Community Health, University of Auckland for providing such a congenial atmosphere in which to work. The preparation of this book was supported by the Scottish Office Home and Health Department and Tayside Health Board.

Chapter 1

INTRODUCTION TO HEALTH SERVICES RESEARCH

INTRODUCTION

One of the first recorded successful treatments, written on a tablet of stone, was by SEKHET'ENANACH, chief physician to one of the Pharaohs around 3000 BC, who *'healed the king's nostrils'* (1). Medicine was also well established early in Chinese civilisation. An early medical textbook, the Pen Tsao (the Great Herbal or Chinese Materia Medica), was written around 3000 BC. A wide range of treatments must also have been in use in the West from an early date, for example the Ebers Papyrus of 1500 BC lists 900 recipes and prescriptions. But the value of this wealth of treatments is in doubt: *'an elaborate pharmacopeia was used but much of the therapy was irrational or ritualistic'* (2). Some of the treatments may have been based on astute clinical observation, although the usefulness of most treatments had not been determined by formal assessment. A common characteristic of early health care is that it was not subjected to systematic research designed to determine whether it was effective.

Medicine in the twentieth century has witnessed an explosion of research. The results of this research have led to understanding, at both the molecular and environmental levels, of the causes of diseases from cancer and heart attacks. They have also led to the development of an impressive array of surgical, pharmacological and rehabilitation therapies. The potential benefits from this research are undoubted; what is less certain is whether they are all being realised in practice: *'a research approach has not been brought to bear systematically on issues relating to the effectiveness of clinical practice, the dispersal and use of existing knowledge, the best use of human and other resources, and the contribution of medical interventions to the health status of individuals and the population'* (3). This range of investigations comes under the banner of health services research.

BACKGROUND TO HEALTH SERVICES RESEARCH

Formal support for medical research in Britain began in 1911, when the Treasury contributed one penny for every person insured under the National Health Insurance Act, amounting to £40 000 in the first year (4). The research policy aimed at *'supporting a wide range and depth of research activities and did not confine itself to specific and urgent health problems'*. But the research has been criticised for not assessing the effectiveness of health care delivery, nor evaluating its quality (5).

A major difficulty facing health services research was *'the absence of a consistent policy for commissioning and funding'* (6). Until recently the situation had changed little; the 1988 report of the House of Lords Select Committee on Medical Research highlighted *'the weakness of health services research'* (7). However, a direct result of the Select Committee's recommendations was the establishment of a National Health Service research and development programme, with an expenditure target of 1.5% of the NHS budget (3). Health services research is now high on the NHS agenda.

DEFINING HEALTH SERVICES RESEARCH

Health services research is one of those unfortunate terms which seem to need no definition; clearly it means research into the delivery of health care. Unfortunately this leaves unanswered exactly what it does and what it is trying to achieve. Health services research comprises many different activities with differing aims and methods. Consider the possibilities for research into the services involved in screening for breast cancer.

Screening for Cancer of the Breast

Breast cancer is the most common form of cancer in women, with 26 000 newly diagnosed cases and 16 000 deaths occurring in Britain each year (8). The case for screening appears attractive because survival from breast cancer improves the earlier the diagnosis is made (9). Early detection through screening should reduce mortality, because the cancers which are detected can be removed by surgery. Two broad research questions arise immediately:

- how good is the screening test?
- does screening work in the community setting?

These broad areas each contain several more specific questions. The value of the screening test will obviously depend on how good it is at detecting early disease and on how many of those who do not have the disease are falsely labelled as having it. But there are other costs to be taken into account, for example the unnecessary further investigations and surgery on women falsely labelled positive (10), as well as the psychological harm caused by the trauma of these procedures (11).

Whether the test works in the community setting is a much more complex issue. In practice women may not attend for screening, or the screening test may not be as discriminating as it was when tested in the laboratory. A general answer to the question of community effectiveness can be obtained by comparing breast cancer mortality among women screened with those not screened. But again there are many other questions which could be asked: Why do some women fail to attend? How could the service be modified to increase uptake? What features of the screening process do not function as well as intended?

Finally there is the question of whether, once established, the service continues to work well in routine practice. The possibility that it might not is raised by the experience with screening programmes for cervical cancer, which in the mid-1980s had a number of defects: *'deaths were occurring that should have been prevented; women had to wait for months for the results of their tests, others were not recalled when they should have been, and many women were still not being screened at all'* (12). The research questions raised here concern the organisation of the systems for calling women to attend and for dealing with positive results and with the accuracy of the interpretation of the test results.

All of these issues were identified when in 1988 the UK National Breast Screening Programme was implemented following the recommendations of the Forrest report (9). Thus from its inception a programme of research and evaluation was planned. This would determine whether a high standard of service was being offered, assess whether the programme was effective, and evaluate whether it provided value for money (13). Even when a new development should work in theory, it still needs to be evaluated in practice.

This example of breast cancer screening shows how an assessment of only a small part of health care, a screening test, can give rise to a whole series of research questions. Clearly, investigations are not limited to the direct clinical benefits of health care. They extend to service organisation, to the assessment of the attitudes, beliefs and motivations of the users and the providers of health care, and to economic evaluation of the care given. Thus health services research is much more than an assessment of how effective is an investigation or treatment: it includes the implications and consequences of the care given for patients and the community as a whole. Health services research is a very broad church.

Defining Health

A significant event in the development of the national health service was the *'alarm at the poor physique of so many of the volunteers for the Boer War (1899–1901)'* (14). Although many other events and individuals were involved, this one is highlighted to emphasise that health care does much more than cure the sick: it aims to produce a healthy population. This is reflected in the World Health Organization definition of health: *'health is a state of complete physical, mental and social well-being and not merely the absence of disease or infirmity'* (15). Although this definition has been criticised (16), it emphasises that health is much more than the absence of illness or disease. The importance of the definition lies in the weight which it gives to well-being, both mental and social as well as physical.

These ideas are reflected in the 1992 White Paper, *The Health of the Nation* (17), whose strategy for improving health describes the twin goals of *'adding years to life . . . adding life to years'*. It is not sufficient to reduce premature death and extend life expectancy. The quality of the life lived should be improved, by minimising the impact of illness and disability and by promoting healthy lifestyles. Health services research is the discipline charged with determining how to achieve this, through improvements in the delivery of health care. A review of the definitions of this branch of research shows how complex this task is.

Definitions of Health Services Research

A number of definitions of health services research have been proposed (Table 1.1). Given the hesitant origins of this branch of research and the scale and complexity of health care systems, it would not be surprising if there were divergent views on the nature of health services research. But there is a remarkable consistency among the definitions listed. They all recognise the breadth of activities involved in health care and hence the variety of types and purposes of research. In general terms, health services research is the discipline which seeks knowledge which will lead to improvements in the delivery of health care.

Table 1.1 Definitions of health services research

Definition	Reference
All strategic and applied research concerned with the health needs of the community as a whole, including the provision of services to meet those needs.	(7)
Scientific activity directed towards the effective and efficient organisation of knowledge, manpower and resources to meet the health needs of a population.	(18)
Research relating to the effectiveness of clinical practice, the dispersal and use of existing knowledge, and the contribution of medical interventions to the health status of individuals and the population.	(19)
It is concerned particularly with the ways in which the distribution, quality, effectiveness and efficiency of health and medical care can be enhanced.	(6)
The investigation of the health needs of the community and the effectiveness and efficiency of the provision of services to meet those needs.	(20)
The identification and quantification of health care needs, and the quantitative study of the provision and use of health services to meet them.	(21)
The evaluation of the adequacy, effectiveness, and efficiency of medical care, including assessments of the need for medical care and of professional and public attitudes.	(22)
The use of the scientific method in investigating problems of planning, organisation and administration (including management and evaluation) of health services.	(23)
The health services research field focuses on the production, organisation, distribution, and impact of services on health status, illness, and disability.	(24)
The study of the scientific basis and management of health services and their effect on access, quality, and cost of health care.	(25)
Health services research studies the health care sector as an organisation, its tasks, resources, activities and results.	(26)

The variety of its activities can be readily seen by listing the areas which health services research can address:

- provision of services
- use of services
- organisation of services
- distribution of services

- quality of services
- planning of services
- health needs of the community
- effectiveness of care
- efficiency of care
- ease of access to services
- equity of use of services
- impact of services on health status, illness and disability
- use of medical knowledge
- attitudes of the public and health professionals

This list comes directly from the terms used in the definitions of health services research, with one exception: equity of use of services. It is curious that this important topic should not feature more prominently, although it is implicit in several of the definitions. The important point is that the list confirms the breadth of health services research and indicates the vast range of topics which could be investigated.

WHY DO HEALTH SERVICES RESEARCH?

In comparison with research into clinical medicine, the delivery of health care has hardly been studied at all. Because it has been largely ignored, health services research has the potential to make a major contribution to health. The value of this research was eloquently argued by Mechanic in 1978: *'To the extent that health services research is done well, it contributes immensely to intelligent policy consideration and more than repays its relatively small investment. . . . a well-structured health services research program is essential to future health care policy and to adequate monitoring of a massive national investment'* (24). A number of different arguments can be put forward to justify the need for research. It is worth reviewing them because they help indicate the range of studies which could be undertaken and what form they should take.

Variations in Health Care

Whenever the health care given in different areas is compared, differences are found in the frequencies with which particular treatments are used. Many studies have confirmed the widespread and persistent variations in a number of surgical operations (27–30). Large differences have also been found in drug prescribing (31), general practitioner referral of patients to outpatient clinics (32, 33) and the use of radiological investigations (34, 35). The implications of these variations are summed up in the title of a paper by a leading American researcher: *'Are hospital services rationed in New Haven or over-utilised in Boston?'* (36). These findings received remarkably little attention until the late 1980s, when commentaries began appearing in leading medical journals (30, 37–40). Whether the explanation is over- or under-treatment, these findings indicate that care is less than optimal.

Inadequacies in Care

The recent prominence given to clinical audit (41) has led to many examples of deficiencies in the quality of care currently being delivered. For example, the Report of a Confidential Enquiry into Perioperative Deaths found that 22% of deaths following surgery were avoidable (42). A separate study found that a larger proportion (61%) of deaths from intussusception in childhood were thought to have avoidable factors (43). Deficiencies have also been reported in the immunization of individuals at high risk of developing hepatitis B (44), in the prescription of thrombolytic treatment to elderly patients with suspected acute myocardial infarction (45), and the excessive use of routine diagnostic tests has been known for over 20 years (46). Many other instances could be listed, for example that inadequate training led to unacceptably high rates of sepsis of intravascular catheters (47) or that the waiting times for routine investigation *'may subject NHS patients to unnecessary risk'* (48). Together these examples illustrate that care can be inadequate in a variety of ways, and that it would be unwise for any professional group to claim that in their province, care is always of the highest standard. Whenever a critical eye has been cast on health care delivery, the potential for improvements in care has been seen. Research is needed to determine how best to identify such deficiencies, and on the strategies which will be most effective at improving care.

Misplaced Medical Models

Many treatments have been based on the prevailing medical models. For example, the doctrine of humours held that disease resulted from an imbalance between the amounts of the four bodily humours. The imbalance was treated by removing some of the one in excess, and so the practice of bleeding was begun. All manner of effective devices were developed for bleeding and any degree of blood loss could be achieved. In some cases, when the patient did not recover, it was assumed that insufficient treatment had been given and additional blood letting was undertaken. It is worth stressing that the practitioners of blood letting passionately believed that their treatment helped the patient.

A more recent example is the use of neuroablative techniques for the treatment of chronic pain. It was thought that pain was transmitted through specific nerve fibres, and interrupting the nerve pathway would therefore relieve the pain (49). Unfortunately, pain sensation is a much more complex phenomenon and there is evidence that neuroablation is not just ineffective, but may even be counterproductive (50). Despite these advances in understanding, many clinicians continue to believe the therapy is of value (51). If medicine is to advance we need to know which models prevail, what evidence they are based on, and the extent to which unjustified models influence the treatments given.

Pace of Innovation

Part of the explanation for inadequacies of care could also be the pace at which innovations are being introduced into medicine. This has been described as 'the "tidal wave" of new technology that was threatening western health-care systems' (52). New techniques may promise improved care, but in practice may not achieve this. For example, there are obvious attractions to using shock wave lithotripsy to smash renal calculi, allowing the resulting fragments to be excreted with the urine. The technique is non-invasive, and might be thought safer and hence a preferable treatment. However, a comparative study found that litho-tripsy was much less effective than percutaneous nephrolithotomy, and surprisingly had a slightly higher complication rate (53). Reservations are also beginning to be expressed about another dramatic innovation, laparoscopic cholecystectomy: 'the uncomfortable conclusion . . . is that the introduction of an attractive new technique has distorted medical practice and overall made care more expensive' (54). Thus, each innovation needs to be evaluated 'to prevent it being adopted merely because it exists rather than because it has been shown to be cost effective' (55).

The pace of innovation carries with it another hazard: that, amid all the other changes taking place, some potentially effective treatments are ignored: 'other technologies were only recognised as effective and adopted more widely after unnecessary and damaging delays: examples include tamoxifen and chemotherapy for early breast cancer, and antiplatelet therapy in cardiovascular disease' (56). The questions for research are why some technologies are rapidly adopted and others are ignored, and what mechanisms need to be in place to ensure that only proven technologies are used.

Unproven Treatments

Many treatments have been shown in clinical trials to be effective and some, when first introduced, were substantial advances on previously best treatments. However, for many treatments currently in use there is no formal evidence that they are effective: *'the plethora of unproven medical practices'* (57). For example, radiotherapy following mastectomy for the treatment of early breast cancer was *'widely advocated for many years . . . without any good evidence for survival benefit'* (58). Eventually an overview of most of the major studies showed *'not only an absence of any survival benefit, but an adverse effect on long-term survival 10 years or more after treatment'* (58).

The recognised method for assessing the efficacy of a treatment is the randomised controlled clinical trial: *'for many forms of care, trials involving sufficient numbers of participants are essential'* (59). A large number of trials are conducted each year, but these are published in a variety of locations. It can be difficult to find them all, and it is not always easy to distil knowledge from the extensive medical literature. To assist busy health professionals the Cochrane Collaboration was established in 1992 to *'assemble and disseminate'* systematic reviews of published studies (59). Health services research must provide the evidence by which health service activities are judged.

Limitation of Resources

Concerns about controlling the extent of spending have been a feature of the NHS since its inception: *'for most of its 43 years, and certainly for the whole of the past quarter century, the dominant issue in the NHS has been its cost . . . it is now widely recognised that public expectations of health care in an affluent society rise consistently and relentlessly'* (60). As well as increased expectations, the cost of medicine inexorably becomes more expensive as new treatments and new methods of investigation are developed: *'the practice of medicine in the twentieth century has grown progressively more dependent on specialized high-technology diagnostic procedures that extend the clinicians' powers of observation'* (61). The consequence of these developments was described by the distinguished American researcher Robert Brook: *'the explosion of costly medical technologies increasingly jeopardises our ability to give everybody all the care that would benefit them'* (62). No matter how willing a community is to pay for health care, decisions will be required on which care to provide and research will be needed to inform these decisions.

Professional Benefits from Research

Health services research is intended to benefit patients and society, by improving health care in the broadest sense. However, there are also direct personal benefits to health professionals from an active involvement in research. These include: the personal satisfaction of contributing to knowledge; the opportunity to change the culture within which health care is delivered by encouraging others to be interested in research; and the potential to improve the nature and quality of the service given. Carrying out research also stimulates interest in reading the literature and hones the critical faculties. Thus it becomes easier to keep abreast of new developments, and to decide which should be incorporated into current practice and which should be left until further studies have been reported.

THE SCOPE OF HEALTH SERVICES RESEARCH

The review of the definitions of health services research (Table 1.1) indicates the very wide scope of research activity to be undertaken. This reflects the breadth of health care: *'health care implies not only the care of the acutely and chronically ill but also rehabilitation, case-finding, health maintenance, prevention of disease and disability, and health education'* (23). This breadth results in a wealth of topics which could be investigated. One way to appreciate the wealth is to recast the definitions of health services research into three questions which can be asked of health care: What resources are available? Which tasks should be performed? What requirements govern the performance of those tasks?

The Resources

The resources of health care are much wider than hospitals and community health centres. They comprise:

- buildings
- equipment
- personnel

When the health service was first formed in 1948 the concerns were whether the staff, buildings and equipment were adequate for the level of care intended; and it quickly became apparent that there was a need for *'a major redistribution of services'* (63). These evident deficiencies were soon remedied, and health services research now investigates more subtle and challenging problems. The question now is whether the health needs of the community are being best met by the balance of resources between the different clinical specialties, and the nature of the provision within specialties. Research is needed to determine the *'volumes and configurations of facilities, personnel, technologies, equipment, and services which will best meet the needs of defined populations within limits imposed by resources and acceptability'* (64, p30). This type of research can be challenging to undertake, involving an overview of health care processes and estimates of the costs and benefits of each service activity. It is much simpler to carry out studies of particular parts of the service, to determine whether they are sufficient to meet the demands being made of them. For example, a survey of the lengths of time patients wait to be seen in outpatients found that *'about half of patients waited more than 3 months for an appointment at a teaching hospital pain clinic; and half waited 9 weeks or longer to be seen at a district general hospital pain clinic. In many clinics the situation is worsening'* (65). The results suggest that additional resources may be required.

The staff who deliver health care are in many ways the most important resource of the health service. It is their training and experience which most directly govern the quality of health care. Health care professionals must be knowledgeable and deliver care with sensitivity and skill. Research has been conducted into all these areas. One study found as expected that doctors' knowledge increased with clinical experience from house officer to senior registrar (66). However, some intermediate grades of doctors overestimated the extent of their knowledge, leading to concern about the ways this could affect their clinical practice. A separate study of cervical screening found several instances where lack of skill and lack of concern about patient anxieties led to unnecessary suffering (67).

Health services research is rightly concerned with what health professionals do, but its scope is much broader. It addresses the issues of the knowledge, attitudes and beliefs and motivations of health care professionals, and how these might be changed to improve care.

The Tasks

The tasks of the health service are to meet the health needs of the individual and the community. These are achieved through three broad strategic objectives:

- promote health
- diagnose and treat disease
- provide care

Promote Health

Promoting good health involves more than just screening to detect disease in its early stages and immunising against infectious disease. It involves empowering individuals to adopt healthy lifestyles and implementing measures to prevent disease. The potential which disease prevention has for improving the health of the nation has been recognised for many years (68). Prevention is particularly attractive because it can be argued that *'the burden of disease and the cost of services could both be reduced by redistributing funds in favour of prevention'* (69). In practice these reductions in cost may not always be realised: *'the evidence . . . shows that, even after allowing for savings in treatment, prevention usually adds to medical expenditures'* (70). The main benefit of prevention is in improving the health of the nation.

For much of the twentieth century prevention was largely neglected, but it is now rapidly moving to centre stage. A seminal role has been played by the World Health Organization's *Health for All* strategy, with its targets for the reduction of disease morbidity and mortality (71). The World Health Organization has also identified research priorities to help achieve its targets (72). In Britain prevention has been given government backing with the publication of targets for disease reduction (17). Research is needed to develop and test health promotion interventions.

Diagnose and Treat

Diagnosis and treatment are often viewed as the central activities of health services. Both are multifaceted. Diagnosis can involve interpersonal skills in interviewing patients, physical examination, use of diagnostic aids ranging from X-rays and laboratory tests to the most up-to-date imaging techniques. Treatments can be equally diverse, ranging from reassurance that there is not a serious underlying disease, through single short-term treatments such as antibiotics for urinary tract infections, to complex multimodal therapy such as drugs, surgery and radiological treatment for cancer. For each step of diagnosis and treatment the research questions to be asked are: Does this work? Is there a need for improvement? What benefits could be gained from alternative approaches? How much would the alternatives cost?

Provide Care

In addition to diagnosing and treating disease, there is a need to care for certain groups of patients. The distinction between treatment and care is highlighted in the management of terminally ill patients. Here the emphasis of management is ensuring as high a level of well-being as possible. Attention is given to the social, psychological and spiritual needs, as well the medical needs of the patient.

There is a need for caring in a number of different situations. For many diseases, rapid cure is not an option. Instead, as with stroke, there may be an extended period of rehabilitation. Even when this process is completed some patients may not be fully recovered, but need longer-term care. For other diseases, like multiple sclerosis, the long-term prognosis is one of disease progression, with increasing disability and handicap leading to increased need for care. The research questions for health care centre on determining what are the most effective and acceptable ways to provide the care. For example, three models for the management of stroke patients have been described by Russell and colleagues: acute units; rehabilitation units; and enhanced home care (73). The concern of the authors of the report was whether *radical changes in existing models of stroke care may incur large costs but bring only small benefits*.

Caring can extend beyond the patient to include their relatives and friends. Those looking after an elderly dementing relative or a dying child are themselves in need of support. There is some recognition of this in the provision of respite care for carers. But the unanswered questions are whether this is sufficient and whether it best meets their needs.

The Requirements

Health care can be summarised as the process by which the health professional delivers care to patients. Health services research addresses each of these three facets of health care—the health professional; the delivery of care; and the well-being of the patient—asking whether there are deficiencies or opportunities for improvement. The overall require-ments of the way health care is delivered is that it should be:

- efficacious
- effective
- efficient
- equitable
- acceptable

The terms efficacious and effective are firmly established in the medical literature. Efficacy is whether an intervention can work (sometimes under ideal conditions), and effectiveness addresses whether it does work in practice. It is perhaps a pity that such similar words were used, but we are stuck with them. The distinction between them can be illustrated with the example of coronary bypass surgery. This operation has been shown in clinical trials to reduce substantially the mortality from left mainstem coronary disease. There is no doubt that it is highly efficacious. But operative mortality is much higher in general use than in the clinical trials, so that overall the treatment is less effective than had been hoped (74). Treatments which work in controlled surroundings on highly selected patients may be less effective in normal clinical practice.

Efficiency refers to value for money. The need for it reflects 'the ubiquitous problem of scarcity in all health care systems' (75). An efficient health care system also concentrates resources 'on those effective services, provided at least cost, that offer the biggest payoff in terms of health' (76). The challenge for research is not just to find ways of delivering effective health care more cheaply, but to identify those areas which will lead to the greatest improvements in health for least cost.

The concept of equity, that all members of the community should have equal access to health care, was woven into the fabric of the NHS when it was established (77). The NHS has an enviable record for providing its service equitably, although in some circumstances this has not been fully achieved. For example, dialysis for end-stage renal disease used to be provided in a way which 'led to the virtual exclusion of patients over the age of 55 years' (78). Discrimination can also occur by sex. Women hospital-ised for coronary heart disease receive fewer investigations and less coronary artery surgery than do men (79, 80). One explanation could be that 'coronary heart disease has traditionally been regarded as a disease of men' (81). Concerns about equity are growing in many countries, including Britain. The issue is regarded with such seriousness in the United States that a 10-year, $500 million research program was established in 1991 (81). There is undoubtedly considerable scope for research on equity in Britain.

Another recent development in the NHS is the increasing awareness that the care given should be acceptable to the patient receiving it. This has become part of national policy since the issuing of Patient's Charters in England, Scotland and Wales in 1991 (82). The intention is to move away from the paternalistic 'doctor knows best' approach to take account explicitly of the patient's views and preferences for treatment (74). There is a growing recognition that patients are capable of making valid judgements of the quality of care which they have received, and that their views should be investigated.

To achieve the five requirements of health care, service delivery should be based on research findings. Research has led to spectacular advances in knowledge in the twentieth century, but it is less clear that the potential benefits for health care have been fully realised. In 1968 Lord Rosenheim addressed the World Health Organization: *'if, for the next twenty years no further research were to be carried out, if there were a moratorium on research, the application of what is already known, of what has already been discovered would result in widespread improvement in world health'* (cited by (83)). The delay in implementation of research findings is as much a feature of current health care as it was nearly 30 years ago (84). It is the province of health services research to explore why these delays occur, and how health professionals can be encouraged to adopt proven new therapies.

WHY HEALTH SERVICES RESEARCH IS DIFFICULT

Research is never easy, but there are a number of factors which conspire to make health services research especially difficult. Although these are not unique to this field, they occur more frequently and with more force than in many other areas of research. The problems are:

- dealing with people
- threat
- measuring outcome
- involving other disciplines
- an educational straitjacket
- time constraints
- lack of control
- ethics

People

The sorts of questions asked in health services research are: Does the use of preoperative chest X-rays lead to improved management of patients? Does a new neuroprotective agent increase survival after a stroke? Does increased dietary calcium reduce the risk of hip fractures in the elderly? These questions focus on important issues of diagnosis, treatment and disease prevention. But in asking these technical questions, the people involved may be overlooked. People are central to the delivery of health care, whether it is the health professionals using the diagnostic equipment or administering therapy, or the patients who receive their attentions. Research into health care inevitably affects these people. This seems reasonable: health care delivery is a multidisciplinary activity, so research into it would be expected to follow suit. To be successful the people who are likely to be affected by the research need to be identified, and involved from the beginning. This is not always easy: *'Handling people is not all that difficult. All you need is inexhaustible patience, unfailing insight, unshakeable nervous stability, an unbreakable will, decisive judgement, irrepressible spirits, a sturdy physique, plus unfeigned affection for all people— and an awful lot of experience'* (85).

The intrusiveness of research can range from a minor irritation to a downright nuisance because daily routine is disrupted. Consider, for example, a project to assess bed use in a psychiatric rehabilitation unit. The interest lay in whether there was inappropriate usage, and hence in the scope for early discharge. This study revealed that almost half of the bed days were taken up by patients who were ready for discharge (86). The study involved all members of the rehabilitation team (consultant, senior registrar, charge nurse, occupational therapist and social worker) in additional patient assessments. It was only possible because all the staff were actively involved in the research from the planning stage. Being involved in a study can generate a sense of ownership of the research, leading to enthusiastic participation.

Threat

As well as being intrusive to health care staff, research can be threatening. At its most extreme a study of the delivery of health care could be likened to an inspector saying: *'We are just going to take a long hard look at your practice to find out what you are doing wrong so that we can make you change.'* Few staff would view a research proposal in this light. But the statement contains two elements which will be felt to some degree: judgement of past performance, and change in care delivery in the future. These need to be recognised and addressed. Anxiety can in part be allayed by emphasising the broader implications of the research: although the study is being conducted locally it is trying to answer questions of much wider importance. Thus it is not trying to find mistakes but to identify ways of meeting the common goal, delivering an even higher quality of service.

Measuring Outcome

The key concern of health care delivery is the resulting outcome for the patient: Did the expected benefit occur? Were there any untoward events? In some circumstances the benefit to the patient may be compelling; as in surgery for prostatic hypertrophy, or H_2 receptor antagonists for duodenal ulcers. For conditions which can be fatal there is a clear measure of the amount of benefit arising. But for many chronic diseases, like asthma or schizophrenia, where death is uncommon, the extent of benefit can be difficult to quantify. The researcher is often forced to use quality of life measures, questionnaire based assessments, to measure the impact of the disease and the benefits of treatment.

Involving Other Disciplines

As already noted, health services research is a very broad church, involving many types of enquiry into all areas of health care. Health services research can be viewed as occupying a central position surrounded by other disciplines and specialties (Figure 1.1). For example, if the research were concerned with planning the nature and extent of renal services it could involve several disciplines: health economics (to address issues of value for money); a combination of public health and information science (to assess the need for services); and operations research (to explore the consequences of following each of the differing options).

Questions commonly asked in health services research are *'Why do people do that?'* and *'What do they think about the service being offered?'* Studies have looked at why doctors prescribe particular drugs (87), why patients fail to keep outpatient appointments (88), what patients think of genitourinary medicine services (89), patient satisfaction with laryngectomy (90), and what visitors think of the care given to elderly patients (91). Teasing out the subtleties of what people believe and the real reasons for particular behaviours is often a feature of health services research. It is also a challenging task. Assessing attitudes and beliefs really falls within the realm of health psychology or medical sociology.

Recognising explicitly when research has moved into another domain means the tools and techniques of that domain can be sought out and used. This is true for the other domains, such as health promotion, medical sociology and health psychology. Each has a well developed theoretical base and a number of practical techniques which can greatly facilitate research.

A second reason for recognising when the research has moved into another domain is to highlight the need for additional expertise. There is

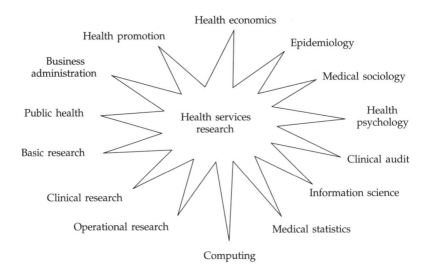

Figure 1.1   Disciplines related to health services research

a wide range of research studies which health professionals can conduct unaided, but many studies will require support from other professionals. Venturing into such studies without this support is akin to wandering round a foreign city without a map or a guide. By some lucky chance you may arrive at the intended destination, but more likely you will become lost and dispirited. Specialists from the appropriate area can not only ensure that the research is done correctly, they will do so far more quickly than the non-specialist could.

An Educational Straitjacket

Medical education *'begins with study of the structure and function of the body (anatomy, physiology, and biochemistry) . . . continues with examination of disease processes (pathology and microbiology); and . . . ends with clinical instruction on selected patients of the types seen in a teaching hospital'* (68). The consequence is to channel thinking towards diagnosis and treatment. There is no encouragement to a critical assessment of wider issues of health care. Students are not trained to ask about the way the service is organised or whether the whole process of care is as effective and efficient as it should be. Students are there to learn about current practice; not to question why it is followed, whether it has a rational basis or simply enshrines tradition. Asking these questions is the role of health services research. Health care professionals need to learn to challenge the way care is organised and delivered.

Time Constraints

The findings from health services research matter because they can lead to improvements in patient care. The corollary is that until the results are available some patients may be suffering unnecessarily. The closer the research is to patient care, the more urgent this time pressure becomes. It is particularly strong when the results are to be used for service planning, when immediate decisions may be wanted. Pressure may be increased because managers *are driven by the need to deliver change in ever shorter timescales* (92). The need to conduct rigorous studies quickly places a substantial extra burden on the design of health services research.

Lack of Control

Much health services research is conducted by observing the way health care is delivered. This is in contrast to laboratory based research where the scientist can control all the factors which might influence the results. Lack of control is a particular problem because *health care delivery is a complex organisational activity* (93). There are myriad factors which can influence the outcome of health care. Thus one of the most common questions in health services research—'why did those events happen?'— can have a large number of possible answers.

The problem of lack of control is particularly marked in studies assessing the impact of changes in service organisation. For example, if a drug formulary is introduced into a hospital, the impact which it has on drug costs could be assessed by comparing costs in periods before and after its introduction. However, other changes could have occurred: a drug company might actively promote one drug; other authoritative guidelines could be issued; changes in referral patterns could result in the treatment of new patients requiring expensive drugs. Because changes inevitably occur over time, it can be difficult to determine how much of the change was due to the intervention and how much to other factors.

When a new service is implemented, for example a day care centre for the elderly or an additional clinic session for childhood immunization, there is often interest in measuring its impact. But unlike a laboratory where experiments can be repeated, in health services research there may only be one opportunity to observe what happened. Thus, if by oversight some important piece of data was not collected, there is no opportunity to do the study correctly a second time.

Ethics

Ethics are of paramount importance in research: *'ethical problems arising from human experimentation have become one of the cardinal issues of our time'* (94). This statement followed a chilling review of dubious research practice involving patients and healthy volunteers. Much health services research does not involve hazardous investigations or treatments, but ethics are still important. The research inevitably imposes on patients' time, and can cause distress. Even simple surveys of patients' knowledge and beliefs about their illness can raise anxieties: about the nature of treatments; or about the long-term prognosis. Any study which involves people, as health services research often does, needs ethical approval from the local research ethics committee. If there is uncertainty about whether ethical permission is required it is better to assume that it will be. Ethical committees act as guardians of patients' rights and can refuse permission for studies, or can request modifications to the design. The obligation to conduct ethical research can increase the complexity of the design and conduct of studies. What is needed are well designed studies of sufficient size (i.e. with a large enough sample of patients) which are able to answer worthwhile research questions with adequate care taken to protect the rights of patients. These designs are not easily achieved.

HOW TO DO HEALTH SERVICES RESEARCH

The review of health services research presented in this chapter shows that it subscribes to the doctrine of the three Ds: diverse, difficult and desirable. It involves a wide-ranging set of activities and faces a number of challenges in addition to those normally encountered in biomedical research. After many years of neglect, the value of health services research has been recognised and a number of initiatives taken at national and regional level to develop this fledgling discipline. The rest of this book explores how to do health services research.

REFERENCES

1. Guthrie, D. *A History of Medicine* (2nd edn). Edinburgh: Thomas Nelson and Sons Ltd, 1958.

2. Bull, JP. The historical development of clinical therapeutic trials. *Journal of Chronic Diseases* 1959; **10**(3): 218–48.
3. Peckham, M. Research and development for the National Health Service. *Lancet* 1991; **338**: 367–71.
4. Dollery, CT. The quality of health care. In: McLachlan, G, ed. *Challenges For Change: Essays on the Next Decade in the National Health Service*. London: Oxford University Press, 1971: 3–32.
5. Bierman, P, Connors, EJ, Flook, E, Huntley, RR, McCarthy, T and Sanazaro, PJ. Health services research in Great Britain. *Milbank Memorial Fund Quarterly* 1968; **46**(1): 9–102.
6. Butler, JR and Boddy, FA. The evolution of health services research in Britain. *Community Medicine* 1983; **5**: 192–9.
7. House of Lords Select Committee on Science and Technology. *Priorities in Medical Research. Volume I: Report.* London: HMSO, 1988.
8. Cancer Research Campaign. Factsheet 6: breast cancer. In: *Facts on Cancer.* London: Cancer Research Campaign, 1991: 1–3.
9. Cancer Research Campaign. Factsheet 7: breast cancer screening. In: *Facts on Cancer.* London: Cancer Research Campaign, 1991: 1–5.
10. Skrabanek, P. The debate over mass mammography in Britain: the case against. *British Medical Journal* 1988; **297**: 971–2.
11. Roberts, MM. Breast screening: time for a rethink? *British Medical Journal* 1989; **299**: 1153–5.
12. Slater, D. National Cervical Screening Programme [editorial]. *British Medical Journal* 1990; **301**: 887–8.
13. Acheson, ED. Breast cancer screening. *Journal of the Royal Society of Medicine* 1989; **82**: 455–7.
14. Leathard, A. *Health Care Provision: Past, Present and Future.* London: Chapman & Hall, 1990.
15. World Health Organization Interim Commission. Constitution of the World Health Organization. *Chronicle of the World Health Organization* 1947; **1**(1–2): 29.
16. Downie, RS, Fyfe, C and Tannahill, A. *Health Promotion: Models and Values.* Oxford: Oxford University Press, 1990.
17. Department of Health. *The Health of the Nation: A Strategy for Health in England.* London: HMSO, 1992.
18. Illsley, R. Research and the NHS. *Health Bulletin* (Edinburgh) 1982; **40**(1): 54–7.
19. Drummond, MF, Crump, BJ and Little, VA. Funding research and development in the NHS. *Lancet* 1992; **339**: 230–1.
20. Medical Research Council. *The Medical Research Council Scientific Strategy.* London: Medical Research Council, 1993.
21. The Wellcome Trust. *Other grants for support of research in health services research and clinical epidemiology.* London: The Wellcome Trust, 1993.
22. Fowkes, FGR, Garraway, WM and Sheehy, CK. The quality of health services research in medical practice in the United Kingdom. *Journal of Epidemiology and Community Health* 1991; **45**: 102–6.
23. Hogarth, J. *Glossary of Health Care Terminology.* Copenhagen: World Health Organization, 1978.
24. Mechanic, D. Prospects and problems in Health Services Research. *Milbank Memorial Fund Quarterly; Health and Society* 1978; **56**(2): 127–39.

25. White, KL. Comments on Navarro's review of *Health Services Research: An Anthology*. *International Journal of Health Services* 1993; **23**(3): 603–5.
26. Bjerregaard, P, Kamper-Jørgensen, F. *Health Services Research in Denmark 1989–1991*. Copenhagen: The Danish Institute for Clinical Epidemiology (DICE), 1992.
27. Wennberg, J, Gittelsohn, A. Small area variations in health care delivery. *Science* 1973; **182**: 1102–8.
28. McPherson, K, Wennberg, JE, Hovind, OB and Clifford, P. Small-area variations in the use of common surgical procedures: an international comparison of New England, England, and Norway. *New England Journal of Medicine* 1982; **307**(21): 1310–14.
29. Jennett, B. Variations in surgical practice: welcome diversity or disturbing differences. *British Journal of Surgery* 1988; **75**: 630–1.
30. Mortensen, N. Wide variations in surgical mortality [editorial]. *British Medical Journal* 1989; **298**: 344–5.
31. Morton-Jones, T and Pringle, M. Explaining variations in prescribing costs across England. *British Medical Journal* 1993; **306**: 1731–4.
32. Wilkin, D and Smith, AG. Variation in general practitioners' referral rates to consultants. *Journal of the Royal College of General Practitioners* 1987; **37**: 350–3.
33. Fowkes, FGR, McPake, BI. Regional variations in outpatient activity in England and Wales. *Community Medicine* 1986; **8**(4): 286–91.
34. Roberts, CJ. Annotation: towards the more effective use of diagnostic radiology: a review of the work of the Royal College of Radiologists Working Party on the more effective use of diagnostic radiology, 1976 to 1986. *Clinical Radiology* 1988; **39**: 3–6.
35. Royal College of Radiologists Working Party. A multicentre audit of hospital referral for radiological investigation in England and Wales. *British Medical Journal* 1991; **303**: 809–12.
36. Wennberg, JE, Freeman, JL and Culp, WJ. Are hospital services rationed in New Haven or over-utilised in Boston? *Lancet* 1987; **i**: 1185–8.
37. Wennberg, J. Which rate is right? [editorial]. *New England Journal of Medicine* 1986; **314**(5): 310–11.
38. Anonymous. Input and outcome [editorial]. *Lancet* 1987; **i**: 1182–3.
39. Dawson, JH. Practice variations: a challenge for physicians [editorial]. *Journal of the American Medical Association* 1987; **258**(18): 2570.
40. Bunker, JP. Variations in hospital admissions and the appropriateness of care: American preoccupations? *British Medical Journal* 1990; **301**: 531–2.
41. Secretaries of State for Health. *Working For Patients*. London: HMSO, 1989.
42. Buck, N, Devlin, HB and Lunn, JN. *Report of a Confidential Enquiry into Perioperative Deaths*. London: Nuffield Provincial Hospitals Trust, 1987.
43. Stringer, MD, Pledger, G and Drake, DP. Childhood deaths from intussusception in England and Wales, 1984–9. *British Medical Journal* 1992; **304**: 737–9.
44. Bhatti, N, Gilson, RJC, Beecham, M, *et al.* Failure to deliver hepatitis B vaccine: confessions from a genitourinary medicine clinic. *British Medical Journal* 1991; **303**: 97–101.
45. Hendra, TJ and Marshall, AJ. Increased prescription of thrombolytic treatment to elderly patients with suspected acute myocardial infarction associated with audit. *British Medical Journal* 1992; **304**: 423–5.
46. Anonymous. Routine diagnostic testing [editorial]. *Lancet* 1989; **ii**: 1190–1.
47. Puntis, JWL, Holden, CE, Smallman, S, Finkel, Y, George, RH and Booth,

IW. Staff training: a key factor in reducing intravascular catheter sepsis. *Archives of Disease in Childhood* 1990; **65**: 335–7.

48. Marber, M, MacRae, C and Joy, M. Delay to invasive investigation and revascularisation for coronary heart disease in South West Thames region: a two tier system? *British Medical Journal* 1991; **302**: 1189–91.

49. Macrae, WA, Davies, HTO and Crombie, IK. Pain: paradigms and treatments [editorial]. *Pain* 1992; **49**: 289–91.

50. Loeser, JD. Ablative neurosurgical operations. In: Bonica, JJ, Loeser, JD, Chapman, CR and Fordyce, WE, eds. *The Management of Pain*. 2nd edn. Philadelphia: Lea & Febiger, 1990: 2040–3. vol II.

51. Davies, HTO, Crombie, IK, Lonsdale, M and Macrae, WA. Consensus and contention in the treatment of chronic nerve-damage pain. *Pain* 1991; **47**: 191–6.

52. Anonymous. Surgical innovation under scrutiny [editorial]. *Lancet* 1993; **342**: 187–8.

53. Mays, N, Challah, S, Patel, S, *et al*. Clinical comparison of extracorporeal shock wave lithotripsy and percutaneous nephrolithotomy in treating renal calculi. *British Medical Journal* 1988; **297**: 253–8.

54. Bateson, M. Second opinions in laparoscopic cholecystectomy. *Lancet* 1994; **344**: 76.

55. Rink, E, Hilton, S, Szczepura, A, *et al*. Impact of introducing near patient testing for standard investigations in general practice. *British Medical Journal* 1993; **307**: 775–8.

56. Health Technology Assessment Advisory Group. *Assessing the Effects of Health Technologies: Principles, Practice, Proposals*. London: Department of Health, 1992.

57. Anonymous. Research and effective health care [editorial]. *Lancet* 1993; **342**: 64–5.

58. Smith, IE. Breast cancer: the qualitative results. In: Bunch, C, ed. *Horizons in Medicine: No. 1*. London: Baillière Tindall, 1989: 305–8.

59. Chalmers, I, Dickersin, K and Chalmers, TC. Getting to grips with Archie Cochrane's agenda [editorial]. *British Medical Journal* 1992; **305**: 786–8.

60. Scotland, A. 25 years of health service change. *British Journal of Hospital Medicine* 1991; **46**: 233–4.

61. Anonymous. Epidemiology and the management of health service resources [editorial]. *International Journal of Epidemiology* 1984; **13**(3): 271–2.

62. Brook, RH. Appropriateness: the next frontier [editorial]. *British Medical Journal* 1994; **308**: 218–19.

63. McLachlan, G. Introduction and perspective. In: McLachlan, G, ed. *A Question of Quality? Roads to Assurance in Medical Care*. London: Oxford University Press, 1976: 3–20.

64. Knox, EG, Acheson, RM, Anderson, DO, Bice, TW and White, KL, eds. *Epidemiology in Health Care Planning: A Guide to the Uses of a Scientific Method*. Oxford: Oxford University Press, 1979.

65. Davies, HTO, Crombie, IK and Macrae, WA. Waiting in pain: delays between referral and consultation in outpatient pain clinics. *Anaesthesia* 1994; **49**: 661–5.

66. Jankowski, J, Crombie, I, Block, R, Mayet, J, McLay, J and Struthers, AD. Self-assessment of medical knowledge: do physicians overestimate or underestimate? *Journal of the Royal College of Physicians London* 1991; **25**(4): 306–8.

67. Crombie, IK, Orbell, S, Johnston, G, Robertson, AJ and Kenicer, M. Women's experiences at cervical screening. *Scottish Medical Journal* 1995; **40**: 81–2.
68. McKeown, T. *The Role of Medicine: Dream, Mirage or Nemesis?* 2nd edn. Oxford: Basil Blackwell, 1979: p 148.
69. Doll, R. Prospects for prevention. *British Medical Journal* 1983; **286**: 445–53.
70. Russell, LB. *Is Prevention Better Than Cure?* Washington, D.C.: The Brookings Institution, 1986. Studies in Social Economics.
71. World Health Organization. *Targets for Health for All: Targets in Support of the European Regional Strategy for Health for All.* Copenhagen: World Health Organization, 1985. European Health for All Series.
72. World Health Organization. *Priority Research for Health for All.* Copenhagen: World Health Organization, 1988. European Health for All Series.
73. Russell, IT, Hamilton, S and Tweedie, V. Models of health care for stroke. *Scottish Medical Journal* 1993; **38**(3 (Supplement)): S15–17.
74. Working Group of the Director of Research and Development of the NHS Management Executive. What do we mean by appropriate health care? *Quality in Health Care* 1993; **2**: 117–23.
75. Maynard, A. Cost management: the economist's viewpoint. *British Journal of Psychiatry* 1993;**163** (Supplement 20): 7–13.
76. Culyer, AJ. The promise of a reformed NHS: an economist's angle. *British Medical Journal* 1991; **302**: 1253–6.
77. Whitehead, M. Who cares about equity in the NHS? *British Medical Journal* 1994; **308**: 1284–7.
78. Kjellstrand, CM and Logan, GM. Racial, sexual and age inequalities in chronic dialysis [editorial]. *Nephron* 1987; **45**: 257–63.
79. Petticrew, M, McKee, M and Jones, J. Coronary artery surgery: are women discriminated against? *British Medical Journal* 1993; **306**: 1164–6.
80. Ayanian, JZ and Epstein, AM. Differences in the use of procedures between women and men hospitalized for coronary heart disease. *New England Journal of Medicine* 1991; **325**(4): 221–5.
81. Khaw K-T. Where are the women in studies of coronary heart disease? [editorial]. *British Medical Journal* 1993; **306**: 1145–6.
82. Stocking, B. Patient's charter [editorial]. *British Medical Journal* 1991; **303**: 1148–9.
83. Kay, AW. *Research in Medicine: Problems and Prospects.* London: The Nuffield Provincial Hospitals Trust, 1977: p75.
84. Smith, R. Filling the lacuna between research and practice: an interview with Michael Peckham. *British Medical Journal* 1993; **307**: 1403–7.
85. Calnan, J. *One Way To Do Research: The A–Z For Those Who Must.* London: William Heinemann Medical Books, 1976: p70.
86. Dick, PH, Crombie, IK, Durham, T, McFee, C, Primrose, M and Mitchell, S. Unnecessary hospitalisation in a psychiatric rehabilitation unit. *British Medical Journal* 1992; **304**: 1544.
87. Bradley, CP. Uncomfortable prescribing decisions: a critical incident study. *British Medical Journal* 1992; **304**: 294–6.
88. Verbov, J. Why 100 patients failed to keep an outpatient appointment— audit in a dermatology department. *Journal of the Royal Society of Medicine* 1992; **85**(5): 277–8.
89. Munday, PE. Genitourinary medicine services; consumers' views. *Genitourinary Medicine* 1990; **66**: 108–11.

90. Jay, S, Ruddy, J and Cullen, RJ. Laryngectomy: the patient's view. *Journal of Laryngology and Otology* 1991; **105**: 934–8.
91. Santamaria, J, Black, J and Knight, PV. Visitors' perceptions of continuing care. *Health Bulletin* (Edinburgh) 1991; **49**(6): 296–8.
92. Roland, M. Getting research into practice [editorial]. *Journal of Epidemiology and Community Health* 1995; **49**: 225–6.
93. McNicol, M, Layton, A and Morgan, G. Team working: the key to implementing guidelines? [editorial]. *Quality in Health Care* 1993; **2**: 215–16.
94. Pappworth, MH. *Human Guinea Pigs: Experimentation on Man.* London: Routledge & Kegan Paul, 1967.

Chapter 2

THE FOUNDATIONS OF RESEARCH

Research can appear intimidating: large laboratories, dedicated scientists and the latest high technology equipment. While some research is of this kind, health services research is usually much less grand and forbidding. It can be as simple as a health care professional asking questions of some patients, where the most important piece of equipment is the sheet of paper to record the answers. It can also involve apparently mundane topics: recent research confirms that inadequate hand washing remains a major cause of hospital-acquired infection (1). Nonetheless, the scientific rigour of health services research can be the equal of that in the best of laboratories, and has the potential to transform fundamentally the way health care is delivered. This chapter provides an overview of what research is, and what it can and cannot do. It introduces reasons for research failing and outlines what can be done to prevent this.

WHAT IS RESEARCH?

Research is a process of finding things out, of filling gaps in our knowledge and understanding of the world. It provides an organised, systematised way of answering questions. It asks *'why this, why not that?'* of the events we see around us. It is a spirit of curiosity encapsulated in a poem from Kipling's *Just So Stories* (2)

'I keep six honest serving men;
(They taught me all I knew);
Their names are What and Where and When
And How and Why and Who.'

For health services research, questions are directed at the organisation and delivery of health care, asking: What is being done? Why is it done that way? How could it be improved? Who is involved in care delivery?

What do I need to find out to understand what is really going on? The last of these questions illustrates a vital step of the research process, clarifying what information is needed to solve the puzzle to hand. Good research asks simple questions which give easily interpreted answers. The questions are not asked in a random or haphazard way. Two of the important skills in research lie in focusing the research questions and fashioning them to provide illuminating answers. The process of doing this is reviewed in Chapter 3.

Because research is meant to provide answers to questions, the research is of little value if it fails to do so. Success does not just refer to the collection of data, but to the provision of useful results. There is an important distinction between data and information. It is easy to gather data: construct and send out a postal questionnaire, or extract items from a set of patient casenotes. It is much harder to gather data which, when analysed, will yield useful information: information that will lead directly to improvements in patient care or the more efficient delivery of that care. The value of a research study is determined by the size and importance of the gap in knowledge which is filled: *the problem must be such that it matters what the answer is'* (3). Value in health services research refers to the potential which the findings have for improving health care. The research findings may not immediately lead to new ways of managing patients or to more efficient or equitable delivery of care. But they should at least clearly point in directions that will lead to these goals.

To plan successful research we need to review what goes on during the research process, and to identify the thinking which underpins the research. In textbooks on the philosophy of science there is much concern with the scientific method. However, many eminent researchers believe that this method is more a construction of philosophers for their benefit than a tool of research: *'Most scientists receive no tuition in scientific method, but those who have been instructed in it perform no better as scientists than those who have not'* (4). Rather than review philosophy, it is more helpful to look at what research does and does not do.

What Research Does

Research involves gathering, analysing and interpreting data to answer the research question. The process may appear glamorous when scientists discuss their findings in television documentaries, but they are presenting in a few minutes the results of many years of work. In reality research can be somewhat mundane, involving great attention to detail, and often requiring the conduct of simple, repetitive tasks.

Before beginning a study you need to clarify its purpose: exactly what you are trying to find out, and what you want the research to achieve. In practice research performs four main tasks. It:

● describes
● searches for explanations
● tests hypotheses
● leads to generalisations

Describing

Much health services research is designed just to find out more about what is going on: *'clinicians and health services researchers have long recognised the poor quality of information on clinical activity in NHS hospitals'* (5). Often quite simple questions are asked: What kinds of patients are being seen? What treatments do they receive? How satisfied are they with their treatment? How many people are there in the community who would benefit from treatment? A study which asked questions like these was carried out by a group who wished to find out more about the patients being seen in an outpatient pain clinic (6, 7). Consultants were asked to complete a short form every time a patient was seen in the clinic. The study produced some unexpected results. For example, there was a substantial delay between being referred and being seen at the pain clinic, and the situation was deteriorating in many clinics; there were marked differences among the clinics in the treatments which were being used. These studies sparked a number of initiatives aimed at improving the quality of care being given (8, 9).

Descriptive surveys, such as that in the pain clinics, are attractively easy to carry out. However, this approach should only be adopted with care, lest it become an exercise in collecting data rather than doing research. In the case of the pain clinic study little previous work had been done in the area, and there was a widespread view among the clinicians that because of professional isolation practice might vary between clinics. A prerequisite for descriptive studies is the hunch—or better, some suggestive evidence—that the findings will be worth the effort of study. Descriptive studies should not be conducted in the hope that something interesting might turn up. Instead they should have clearly defined aims and be focused on an area with an acknowledged paucity of information. There should be a high degree of expectation that the efforts of research will be justified by the wealth of the findings.

Searching

The natural extension to describing how health care is delivered is to search for the reasons for events occurring as they do. The wide-ranging nature of these studies can be seen from the titles of published papers: How elderly patients with femoral fracture develop pressure sores in hospital (10); Outpatients: can we save time and reduce waiting lists? (11); Which tasks performed by pre-registration house officers out of hours are appropriate? (12); Can out of hours work by junior doctors in obstetrics be reduced? (13); Why 100 patients failed to keep an outpatient appointment (14).

Descriptive and exploratory studies ask different types of question. Descriptive studies help clarify what is going on: the what, where and when of Kipling's honest serving men. Exploratory studies extend this investigation to look for reasons: the how, why and who. The implication is that by finding out why events occur, something can be done to alter them. Altering can refer to a number of different actions: curtailing ineffective or wasteful activities; encouraging neglected or overlooked activities; providing education programmes; changing clinic organisation. The more the study has probed why events happen as they do, the more likely that effective action can be taken to improve the efficiency and quality of care.

Testing

Research often involves testing hypotheses. In health services research hypotheses are statements about health care. They attempt to explain why certain events have happened, or to predict what will happen in the future. Hypotheses may concern the way care is organised and delivered, or the effects it has on patients' well-being, or even about the way patients behave. Examples of hypotheses are:

- elderly patients with stroke receive less attention than younger stroke patients;
- delays in obtaining the results of biochemical tests cause an unnecessary increase in the length of in-patient stay;
- patient satisfaction predicts compliance with therapy.

The important feature of these hypotheses is that they can be tested because they make predictions. The above examples make different predictions about: the amount of care given; a factor which determines length of stay; and a factor which influences compliance with therapy. Each of these hypotheses provides an unambiguous statement for testing and specifies the type of data which should be collected. For example, a study of stroke patients might observe the number and length of contacts between patients and health care staff, to test whether older patients do receive less attention. The feature of testing provides us with a means of assessing the value of hypotheses: a good hypothesis is one whose prediction can be easily tested. Once it has been tested by observation we are faced with two choices. The data may not support the hypothesis so it must be discarded. The benefit of this is that, once it has been discarded, some other idea can be investigated instead. Alternatively, the data may be found to be consistent with the hypothesis, so that it cannot be rejected. This does not mean that the hypothesis is true: there may be other tests which it may fail, or it may be modified by subsequent observation. It remains simply as a working hypothesis.

There are other features which contribute to a good hypothesis. For example, the statement that postgraduate educational programmes achieve success by a generalised increase in awareness (rather than, say, by conveying specific pieces of knowledge) is a poor hypothesis. It is difficult to measure generalised awareness. In general hypotheses are poor if:

- they make no real predictions;
- the predictions which they make cannot be measured;
- the study required to test the predictions is unethical;
- the resources required for the study are unlikely to be forthcoming.

Good hypotheses describe the relationship between specific measurable factors. Thus the hypothesis that the quality of nursing care determines the time until full recovery becomes much more easily testable when the important components of quality of care and the measure of recovery are defined.

From Describing to Searching to Testing

There is an implied logical sequence moving from describing what is going on, to seeking the reasons why events occur, to testing whether the proposed explanations for events actually work in practice. It might be tempting to pretend that research follows this logical course, with observations leading inexorably to the testing of ideas. Research seldom proceeds this way. The delivery of care may be described, but the reasons for deficiencies are often not sought. Hypotheses may result from a flash of insight, rather than from a period of exploration. However, the logical route from observation to experiment becomes important when developing a research idea. It emphasises that it is not enough just to look to see what is happening. It encourages attempts to uncover the reasons for events occurring, and the testing of the validity of these ideas. The process of clarifying and refining research ideas is more fully developed in Chapter 3.

Generalising

Whether research is aimed at describing what is going on or testing hypotheses, the hope is that the findings can be generalised beyond the narrow circumstances in which the study was conducted. Consider the finding that substantial numbers of bed days in one particular acute psychiatric ward are being taken up by patients who should be discharged (15). The implications of this are much greater if it can be assumed that similar findings would be made in other acute wards. The value of the research depends on the relevance which it has for other institutions, on the extent to which it can be generalised.

The need for generalisable research has important implications for the design of research studies. Its most important effect is on the choice of subjects to be studied. Suppose that a new model for the rehabilitation of stroke patients is to be tested. There would be little point in testing the new service on a highly selected and atypical set of patients. The more representative the group is of stroke patients in general, the more widely the model can be applied in practice (if it is found to be effective). However, there are constraints on this: for example, the proposed rehabilitation service might be more effective for those who were less severely affected. Thus the patient group to be studied would have to be restricted to these patients to maximise the chances of detecting whether the new service is effective. The challenge is to define as broad a group of patients as possible which is compatible with the supposed therapeutic effect.

Concern about the representativeness of the group being studied applies whatever type of health services research is being carried out. If the group being studied is unusual, the findings may not be widely applicable. It is a useful discipline when designing a study to specify explicitly the wider group to whom the findings are to be extrapolated.

What Research Does Not Do

The research process is a powerful force for advancing our knowledge, but there are things it cannot do and does not try to do. Research does not:

- seek proof
- give guarantees

Research does not try to seek proof. This is in part because proving that an idea is correct can be very difficult, but also because the process of seeking proof can be misleading. The difficulty of obtaining proof can be seen by considering the statement: all ravens are black. It would be extremely tedious and unthinkably expensive to prove the statement by inspecting every raven to determine its colour. Even if a substantial number of ravens had been seen and all were black, this does not mean that all the remaining ones are also black. The statement cannot easily be proved by observation. But suppose a single raven is found to be white. The statement is immediately shown to be false. In general, it is much easier to show a hypothesis to be false. The testing of a hypothesis involves giving it the opportunity to show itself to be false. If a hypothesis makes a prediction which does not occur, then we can refute the hypothesis. But if the prediction turns out to be correct this does not prove the hypothesis to be true. It might have withstood one test, but there may be another which it will fail. For example, Newton's theory of gravitation passed all tests until Einstein's theory of relativity suggested some novel tests which it was unable to pass.

The danger of trying to prove a hypothesis correct was highlighted in a recent whimsical paper on the nature of evidence and scientific proof. It began with the hypothesis that carrying an umbrella gave protection against attacks by lions (16). This was based on the author's observation that he had never been attacked while carrying one. In order to prove this contention, 298 reports of lion attacks were reviewed to determine how many of those who were attacked had been reported as carrying an umbrella. None had. Further support for the idea was adduced from direct observation of 2241 Christians who were carrying umbrellas, the observations were made on Sunday mornings as people were leaving churches. None were under lion attack. The fallacy behind this whimsy is that the evidence would only have value if persons known to be carrying umbrellas were in close proximity to lions and thus liable to attack. Any amount of evidence on persons who were attacked in circumstances where umbrellas would not normally be carried, or where umbrellas were carried but there was no risk of attack, tells us nothing about the validity of the hypothesis.

A further feature of research is that there is no guarantee that a particular study's findings are correct. Newspaper reports of scientific discoveries often claim that researchers have proved, for example, that human beings originated in East Africa, or that coffee causes pancreatic cancer. Sometimes individual claims are subsequently challenged by the findings of further studies. It is not uncommon for new studies to challenge the findings of previous ones, or for cherished theories to be abandoned because they are shown to be incomplete or inadequate. Research provides evidence from which conclusions may be drawn, but the evidence may be faulty or the logic of the conclusion may be flawed. Research findings should be treated with caution, as even the most convincing may be wrong.

The strength of evidence is increased when more than one study reports similar findings, but this still does not mean the conclusions are correct. For example, three studies published in a single issue of the journal *Lancet* all showed that reserpine, a drug which was used for the management of hypertension, increased the risk of developing breast cancer (17). They were accompanied by an editorial which suggested that some patients who were receiving this effective drug should have their treatment suspended. Subsequently a further nine studies were published which failed to show any association between the drug and the risk of cancer. The initial suggestion of a causal association is now thought to be incorrect. The original findings were most likely due to methodological flaws (18).

Fortunately, it is very unusual for research findings to be so misleading. But it must be borne in mind that some studies are better in design and execution than others. All new studies should be reviewed critically and their findings accepted only when there is reliable and compelling evidence (see Chapter 4 on the critical assessment of published papers).

What Research Seldom Does

The previous two sections provided guidance on what research does and does not do. There are other features of research which, although they may occur, rarely do. Research seldom:

- goes smoothly
- revolutionises understanding
- gives clear-cut findings
- contains no surprises

Research often provides support for Murphy's law: *'if something can go wrong it will.'* It has been said that research goes through six stages (provenance unknown):

1. Initial excitement
2. Disillusionment
3. Panic
4. Searching for the guilty
5. Punishing the innocent
6. Honour and praise for the non-participants

Everyone involved in research has experienced stage 1, and most experience 2 and 3. However, comparatively few studies end with honour or praise for anyone, let alone the main participants. This may appear a jaundiced view, but in health services research there are numerous ways in which difficulties can arise. Respondents to questionnaires will find ingenious ways to misunderstand questions and thus give inappropriate answers. Information which should have been recorded in casenotes will be missing, and many of the casenotes themselves will remain stubbornly unavailable. The photocopier will break the very day you need to make 100 copies of the patient information leaflet. Groups of patients who were previously common in clinics will mysteriously become rare as soon as it is decided to study them. The statistician who agreed to help with the study design and analysis will suddenly move to a new job in southern California. The only way to deal with problems is to expect that some mishaps will occur. Thus each stage of a study should be tried out before beginning the definitive study. It is also helpful to build some leeway into the study timetable so that the occasional mishap does not ruin the whole project. Far better to have a few months spare at the end of a study, time which can used to write up the findings or to plan the next study, than to fail to finish a project because of one or two unforeseen difficulties.

There is a view that research questions need to be clever and profound, with answers which will revolutionise our understanding of disease and lead to substantial improvements in patient care. It would be wonderful to carry out such studies, but even the most able and gifted researchers seldom do so. The major advances in medicine, for example the developments of penicillin or thrombolytic therapy for myocardial infarction, are notable for being rare. Almost all medical research produces only small steps forward in our understanding of disease or the delivery of health care. A study which led to even a modest improvement in patient care would be viewed as the crowning achievement in the career of any researcher. A simple study which is well carried out will always be viewed by other researchers as a major achievement.

The interpretation of research findings is sometimes clear cut. For example, a comparison of two management regimes for patients with persistent anxiety showed that one was substantially better (19); and an assessment of the economic impact of early discharge for hip fracture patients showed that there were lower direct costs of rehabilitative care (20). But in other instances findings of research studies can be difficult to interpret. A cursory inspection of the papers published in leading medical journals will show that conclusions of the form *'these findings show . . .'* are not common. Instead conclusions are often couched in more careful language: *'there is an association between quality of intra- partum care and death'* (21); *'these results suggest that haemorrhoids in patients with excessive activity of the internal anal sphincter are best treated by anal dilatation'* (22). Careful words like association, suggest and support are forced upon authors because the findings of studies into health care can be influenced by many factors other than those being studied.

One of the joys of research is that when data are collected and analysed something unexpected often pops out. Some of the findings may be as predicted, but there may a subtle twist to the results. For example, a clinical trial was undertaken to test the belief that sedation helps in fibreoptic bronchoscopy (23). It showed that doctors could carry out the procedure much more easily in sedated patients, and both doctors and nurses thought it more comfortable for the patients. However the patients themselves did not find it more comfortable, and were less willing to have the test repeated if they had been sedated. This propensity of studies to offer glimpses of the unexpected is a reward for the careful researcher.

The Role of Theories

Theories abound in research. They have three useful properties: they describe the way things are; they predict what might happen in different circumstances; and they encourage speculation about the way things might be. For example, the theory that the earth is flat is a description of the earth which predicts that sailors venturing to its edge would be in danger of falling off. This theory also encourages speculation about what supports the flat surface and what exists beyond its edges. A theory is much broader in scope than a hypothesis, which also predicts, because it contains the explanation for the prediction. Thus the prediction follows logically from the theory.

Theories play an important role in medicine. The theories we hold about the pathology of disease direct our thoughts about whether treatments should work. For example, the view of pain proposed by Descartes was that stimulation of specific nerves led to the sensation of pain in the brain. According to the theory painful conditions could be treated by interrupting nerve pathways, and a number of neurolytic techniques were developed (24). However, observations over the first half of the twentieth century of patients with pain showed that this theory was unsatisfactory; pain is a much more complex phenomenon involving a sophisticated processing of all sensory information. According to the new theory of pain, the gate control theory, cutting nerves could be ineffective and could even make the pain worse. This new theory also successfully predicted that stimulation analgesia would be a useful treatment for certain types of chronic pain.

Theories can influence the way health care is organised. For example, it is widely accepted that the more often a procedure is carried out the more skilfully it is done (25): the more operations a surgeon carries out the higher the success rate. This leads to increased specialisation and to particular operations being carried out in regional centres rather than in all hospitals. The trend has been seen most recently in vascular surgery, where specialist surgeons achieve substantially better results. Thus it has been recommended that each health region in Britain should have four to six vascular units each comprising three to four vascular surgeons (26).

Because theories influence speculation they can also affect the nature of the research which is carried out. The germ theory of disease leads naturally to the search for antibiotics. Similarly, there is a general view that in its early stages cancer is a local disease which only becomes systemic later. This theory encourages the development of screening tests to detect asymptomatic disease, and supports the localised use of radiotherapy. Acceptance of the iceberg phenomenon, that diseases known to general practitioners represent only the tip of the iceberg of that disease which exists in the community (27), leads to assessment of the extent of unmet need for medical care in the wider community.

The Dangers of Theories

The obvious danger of theories is that they can be wrong. It is easy for us to look at the discarded theories of the past and recognise the follies that follow from them. What is more challenging is to anticipate which of our current theories will fall into disrepute, as new evidence is uncovered.

Knowing that a theory is being used to organise health care or to plan research means that its validity can be reassessed when new information emerges. However most of us have theories of our own on how health care should be organised and delivered, and what should be done to improve care. Often these theories are not stated explicitly, although they will influence our thinking and the types of research we plan. Thus when identifying topics for research, it can be helpful to ask not only: Why are things done that way? but also to ask oneself: Why do I think this way?

TYPES OF UNSUCCESSFUL RESEARCH

Not all research studies meet with success. Although good or bad luck can influence the course of a project, the outcome is often predictable. There is truth in the Old Testament proverb: '*As ye sow, so shall ye reap.*' Depending on the amount of planning that went into the design and the care taken in the execution, research studies can meet with a variety of unfortunate fates. They can be:

- fatally flawed
- uncompleted
- unpublished
- repetitious
- dull
- ignored

Fatally Flawed

In general all studies contain some defects, perfection being unattainable. Some studies contain such serious flaws that their results are worthless. But it is usually possible to eliminate the major flaws which render the findings uninterpretable, provided the design is subject to severe critical assessment before the study is undertaken. The essence of good study design is adequate planning and ruthless self-criticism. This not only leads to better studies, it also deprives the armchair critics of the pleasure of ravaging your results.

Uncompleted

Perhaps the most common fate of research projects is that they are never completed. This can occur because the study was more difficult than was initially thought, or because it required skills and expertise which the researchers did not have. In addition to adequate planning, the components of a study need to be tried out before beginning the research in earnest. Only when they have been piloted and found to work, or suitably modified if they have failed, should the main study be commenced. The guiding rule is: *'Do not begin unless you are sure you can finish.'*

Unpublished

Many studies are completed but are never published, and their results languish unseen in filing cabinets. A common explanation is that no one had set aside the time to finish the data analysis, prepare the tables and graphs, and write and revise the manuscript. The enthusiasm for a project has usually worn very thin by the time it comes to writing reports, and it can take great effort and perseverance to see it through to publication. The planning of a new study can seem much more interesting than soldiering away at the wearisome task of writing the final report of a completed one. Successful research requires self-discipline.

Repetitious

New ideas for projects are rare, and it may happen that someone has already published a study similar to the one you had in mind. This may not matter because the findings from a single study are often tentative, requiring confirmation by further research. However, if the results are already well established then repetition is pointless. A literature review needs to be conducted before a study is undertaken.

Dull

The fate of all too many studies is to be met with the greeting *'Oh yes, but so what?'* The 'so what?' response is evoked because, although the findings may be new, they are thoroughly uninteresting. This may occur because the results are only relevant to local circumstances. For example, studies of the last 50 patients may seem important to the clinician who saw them, but no one else may care very much. Dull studies can be avoided by asking: *'What implications could the findings have for others?'*

Ignored

A sad fate for a study is for the published paper which comes from it to disappear without trace: no one requests reprints and it is never cited in subsequently published papers. This can happen when the paper is published in the wrong journal, one which is not often read by those you wish to influence. For example, a paper on the psychological consequences of chronic pain could well be published in one of the journals specialising in pain. If so, it is unlikely to be read by many psychologists and would be unlikely to be cited in psychology journals. Similarly, a paper on the epidemiology of coeliac disease published in an epidemiology journal is unlikely to be read by the clinicians who treat this disease. The way to avoid being ignored is to identify the audience that you want to reach and then publish in the journals they read. The same principle applies to presenting papers at conferences. Dissemination of the findings should be seen as an integral part of a project. A good study will involve the identification of the people who should be influenced, and should seek the best ways of doing this. An element of good design is ensuring that results will not be ignored.

The foregoing discussion has shown that a variety of reasons can conspire to make research unsuccessful. The common theme linking these reasons is that important tasks are given insufficient attention or are completely ignored. Research is difficult, but it is more likely to be successful if you:

- critically assess the design
- pilot
- assess the costs, resources and expertise required
- read the literature
- plan
- assess potential benefits

Carrying out each of these activities will help to ensure successful research. Good research projects share certain characteristics, and it is helpful to review them.

CHARACTERISTICS OF A GOOD RESEARCH PROJECT

There is no guarantee that any project, no matter how well planned, will produce exciting findings. But attention to some key issues will help ensure that the study will work, and the findings will be of interest. These issues are:

- soluble problems
- realistic aims
- important issues

Soluble

Research was described as *'the art of the soluble'* by Peter Medawar, a leading scientist of his day. He commented: *'No scientist is admired for failing in the attempt to solve problems that lie beyond his competence. . . . Good scientists study the most important problems they think they can solve'* (28). Before beginning a study the researcher should have a pretty shrewd idea that it will be successful in producing an answer. This doesn't mean that the study will always yield a startling new finding. Often studies have negative findings, showing that what at the time seemed reasonable in fact is not the case. Research often involves *'going up alleys to see if they are blind'* (29). The important point is that the study is concluded and an answer obtained.

One way of looking at solubility is to ask *'Can we get a handle on this problem?'* That is, can we find some way of approaching it that will tell us more about what is going on. To take another analogy, solving a research question is like trying to open a Brazil nut. Biting it would probably break a few teeth, and hitting it with a hammer would smash the nut inside. Careful reflection on a problem will often uncover the appropriate metaphorical nut cracker.

Realistic

An issue separate from whether a question is soluble is whether the study which would be required to solve it is realistic. The distinction is between having a research design which could answer the research question and having the resources required for that design. A common problem is to be overambitious and design a study so that *'a twenty-year research program would be required in order to realize the stated objectives'* (30). Resource does not just refer to money, but to all the materials needed to complete the study, including staff with appropriate expertise, patients, filing cabinets and computers.

Unrealistic studies arise because research issues are often complex and many different questions could be asked. But ambitious wide-reaching studies have a habit of collapsing under their own weight. By trying to answer several questions at once, they end up answering none. Often the methodology used to answer the many questions of the ambitious study is an unhappy compromise between the conflicting requirements of the several aims.

The danger of trying to answer too many questions is magnified when collaborative studies are undertaken. Each collaborator may have specific issues which they want investigated, and suggest additional data items to be collected. In practice only a few questions can be asked at one time, so the most important objectives need to be identified and clearly stated: *'to avoid an unhappy compromise that is adopted in the hope of pleasing everybody'* (30).

Realistic studies are often focused on a very limited part of health care. The appropriate research method will be clear and only a limited amount of data will be collected. If it has been carefully designed clear-cut answers should emerge. Perhaps equally important, focused studies can be completed more quickly, hopefully before the researcher's enthusiasm fades.

Identifies Important Issues

The need for realism does not mean that research has to be dull. Instead, this emphasises the importance of picking a worthwhile topic. Even in a highly specialised research field there are more than enough topics to keep a team of researchers busy for a lifetime. The challenge is to select those which will give the greatest advance with the least effort. A good example is the unravelling of the structure of DNA. Two researchers, Francis Crick and James Watson, had decided that this was the central problem in molecular biology, and for solving it they were subsequently awarded the Nobel prize. They modestly confess that *'by blundering about we stumbled on gold'* (31), but that was no accident: they were looking for gold. Few researchers would expect to gain this pre-eminence, but all can avoid studying dull problems: *'dull or piffling problems yield dull or piffling answers'* (3).

Successful research begins with a good research question. The next chapter reviews ways of identifying those questions.

REFERENCES

1. Jarvis, WR. Handwashing—the Semmelweis lesson forgotten? *Lancet* 1994; **344**: 1311–12.
2. Kipling, R. *Just So Stories*. New York: Airmont Publishing Company, 1966.
3. Medawar, PB. *Advice to a Young Scientist*. New York: Harper & Row, 1979: p13.
4. Medawar, P. *Pluto's Republic*. Oxford: Oxford University Press, 1982: p78.
5. Black, N. Information please—and quick. *British Medical Journal* 1989; **298**: 586–7.

6. Crombie, IK and Davies, HTO. Audit of outpatients: entering the loop. *British Medical Journal* 1991; **302**: 1437–9.
7. Davies, HTO, Crombie, IK, Macrae, WA and Rogers, KM. Pain clinic patients in northern Britain. *The Pain Clinic* 1992; **5**(3): 129–35.
8. Davies, HTO, Crombie, IK and Macrae, WA. Why use a pain clinic? Management of neurogenic pain before and after referral. *Journal of the Royal Society of Medicine* 1994; **87**: 382–5.
9. Davies, HTO, Crombie, IK, Macrae, WA, Charlton, JE and Rogers, KM. *Audit in Pain Clinics: gaining commitment to change.* Clinical Resource and Audit Group, 1994.
10. Versluysen, M. How elderly patients with femoral fracture develop pressure sores in hospital. *British Medical Journal* 1986; **292**: 1311–13.
11. Duncan, M, Beale, K, Parry, J and Miller, RA. Outpatients: can we save time and reduce waiting lists? *British Medical Journal* 1988; **296**: 1247–8.
12. McKee, M, Priest, P, Ginzler, M and Black, N. Which tasks performed by pre-registration house officers out of hours are appropriate? *Medical Education* 1992; **26**: 51–7.
13. McKee, M, Priest, P, Ginzler, M and Black, N. Can out-of-hours work by junior doctors in obstetrics be reduced? *British Journal of Obstetric Gynaecology* 1992; **99**: 197–202.
14. Verbov, J. Why 100 patients failed to keep an outpatient appointment— audit in a dermatology department. *Journal of the Royal Society of Medicine* 1992; **85**(5): 277–8.
15. Dick, PH, Crombie, IK, Durham, T, McFee, C, Primrose, M and Mitchell, S. Unnecessary hospitalisation in a psychiatric rehabilitation unit. *British Medical Journal* 1992; **304**: 1544.
16. Anderson, DR. Umbrellas and lions. *Journal of Clinical Epidemiology* 1991; **44**(3): 335–7.
17. Labarthe, DR. Methodologic variation in case-control studies of reserpine and breast cancer. *Journal of Chronic Diseases* 1979; **32**: 95–104.
18. Horwitz, RI and Feinstein, AR. Exclusion bias and the false relationship of reserpine and breast cancer. *Archives of Internal Medicine* 1985; **145**: 1873–5.
19. Dick, PH, Sweeney, ML and Crombie, IK. Controlled comparison of day-patient and out-patient treatment for persistent anxiety and depression. *British Journal of Psychiatry* 1991; **158**: 24–7.
20. Hollingworth, W, Todd, C, Parker, M, Roberts, JA and Williams, R. Cost analysis of early discharge after hip fracture. *British Medical Journal* 1993; **307**: 903–6.
21. Gaffney, G, Sellers, S, Flavell, V, Squier, M and Johnson, A. Case-control study of intrapartum care, cerebral palsy, and perinatal death. *British Medical Journal* 1994; **308**: 743–50.
22. Keighley, MRB, Buchmann, P, Minervini, S, Arabi, Y and Alexander-Williams, J. Prospective trials of minor surgical procedures and high-fibre diet for haemorrhoids. *British Medical Journal* 1979; **2**: 967–9.
23. Hatton, MQF, Allen, MB, Vathenen, AS, Mellor, E and Cooke, NJ. Does sedation help in fibreoptic bronchoscopy? *British Medical Journal* 1994; **309**: 1206–7.
24. Macrae, WA, Davies, HTO and Crombie, IK. Pain: paradigms and treatments [editorial]. *Pain* 1992; **49**: 289–91.
25. Luft, HS, Hunt, SS and Maerki, SC. The volume–outcome relationship:

practice makes perfect or selective referral patterns? *Health Service Research* 1987; **22**(2): 157–82.

26. Michaels, JA, Galland, RB and Morris, PJ. Organisation of vascular surgical services: evolution or revolution? *British Medical Journal* 1994; **309**: 387–8.
27. Last, JM. The iceberg: "completing the clinical picture" in general practice. *Lancet* 1963; **ii**: 28–31.
28. Medawar, PB. *The Art of the Soluble.* Harmondsworth: Penguin Books, 1969: p11.
29. Bates, M. In: Green J, ed. *A Dictionary of Contemporary Quotations.* London: Pan, 1982: 217.
30. Cochran, WG and Cox, GM. *Experimental Designs* 2nd edn. New York: John Wiley & Sons, 1957: p10.
31. Crick, F. *What Mad Pursuit.* London: Penguin, 1990: p74.

Chapter 3

DEVELOPING THE RESEARCH QUESTION

The kernel of any study is the research question. But this raises a number of uncertainties: Where do the questions come from? How do I know it is a good research question? Can I realistically expect to find the answer? Is the answer worth the trouble? These are the issues which this chapter addresses. It reviews the process of developing the research question, beginning with the original idea, then clarifying the nature of the problem, and finally producing a worthwhile, researchable question. The difficulty of describing this process is that there are no formal rules which can be listed. The process can be introduced with an example.

IDENTIFYING THE RESEARCH QUESTION: AN EXAMPLE

Background to Chronic Pain

Chronic pain is a major public health problem. An estimated 5 million people in the United Kingdom suffer unrelieved pain lasting longer than three months (1). Chronic pain can be severe and debilitating, and is often challenging to treat. Management is difficult because pain can embrace many different dimensions. These include the intensity and quality of pain, and the patients' affective and behavioural response to their pain (2, 3). Chronic pain patients are often managed in outpatient pain clinics (1), and for many cure is not a realistic option. The pain clinic approach is aimed at maximising social, psychological and physical function (4).

The Initial Question

The source of the research question was, as is often the case, clinical experience. Pain clinicians often ask how much good are pain clinics doing, with the implicit aim of identifying ways in which care could be improved. A similar question could be asked of any branch of medicine. *'Can this question form the basis of a worthwhile research project?'*

Assessing the Question

The initial evaluation of the question focused on three areas: the potential implications of the study; the type of study design required; and the resource implications of the study. Chronic pain is a major problem, where even small improvements in management would be worthwhile. Because there is a high degree of interest among pain clinicians in the question, it is likely that any findings would be adopted into clinical practice.

Attention now turns to specifying in more detail how the study could be carried out. One approach would be to compare the outcome of patients attending the clinic with a similar group who did not attend. This could be achieved by identifying new referrals to the pain clinic and randomly assigning them either to be treated at the clinic or to be sent back untreated to the referring physician. Obviously such a study would be unethical. A second problem concerns the resource implications of measuring the benefit to patients from attending the clinic. There are standard questionnaires for assessing social, psychological and physical health, but each takes time to administer and collecting these data could intrude into clinic routine. This could affect the willingness of clinicians to take part.

One solution to the intrusiveness of data collection would be to use self-administered questionnaires. An extension of the self-administered questionnaire would be to develop a computer-administered questionnaire. There is evidence that patients can successfully use computers in this way, and that they may even prefer to answer questions on a computer screen than to fill in paper questionnaires.

An additional benefit of computerised data collection is that it would be possible to process and summarise the data instantaneously. Ordinarily the questionnaires would be coded, the summary score calculated and evaluated; a time-consuming business. In contrast, a computer could provide the clinician with the summary score together with guidance on its interpretation almost as soon as the patient has finished typing in the answers.

An Alternative Question

The suggestion of using a computer for data collection sparked an alternative research question: What would be the effect on patient management of giving the doctor immediate feedback of information from the questionnaires? This could be made the subject of an ethical study. Data would be collected on all patients, but for only half (randomly selected) would it be provided to the clinician. Thus the intervention group would have the benefit of the additional information while the controls would enjoy current best management. The attraction of this design is that it focuses on improving the management of chronic pain. In addition, it would provide information on the extent to which pain patients have psychosocial problems and could thus be used by the pain clinics to argue for additional resources.

At this stage attention was given to finding out whether a study asking this question had been carried out before. A literature review quickly revealed that, although the approach had been used in other specialties, it had not been evaluated within pain. The next question was whether the study was feasible.

Assess the Practicability

The practicability of the study depended on whether sufficient patients could be recruited and whether the necessary data could be collected. An initial sample size calculation indicated that no single clinic could provide sufficient patients, and in the event three clinics would be required. A research coordinator would also be needed to develop the data collection system and to teach and encourage clinic staff to use the computer. Thus substantial research funds would have to be sought to carry out the project.

The example shows that the process of obtaining a researchable question can be divided into a number of stages:

- having an idea
- stating the research question
- refining the research question
- reviewing the literature
- assessing the practicability

Although these stages are given as a list, the example showed that they need not be carried out in sequence. In practice, progress will gradually be made in each stage and the results of efforts in one may influence the others.

HAVING THE IDEA

A few exceptional scientists have inspired ideas. A celebrated example was Archimedes who, according to legend, was lying in his bath when he was struck by a method of measuring the volume of solids through the amount of water they displace. So excited was he by the idea that he rushed through the streets naked, shouting 'Eureka, Eureka' (I have found it). For most of us, ideas for research projects have less dramatic origins.

Reports of published studies often present a logical development for their research. For example, Gaffney and colleagues (5) chose to study the relationship between the quality of obstetric care and the development of cerebral palsy because of the on-going debate on the issue. But it is difficult to be sure which is the most common source of ideas for projects, because scientific papers *not only merely conceal, but actively misrepresent the reasoning that goes into the work they describe* (6). There is a natural tendency to indulge in a touch of *post hoc* rationalisation and describe a study as a logical development from previous work. The more realistic but prosaic explanations like *'I had an argument with a colleague about it'*, or *'I never really understood why we followed that routine'*, are seldom mentioned. Whatever the truth of the matter, there are a number of strategies which can help foster research ideas:

- review existing practice
- challenge accepted ideas
- look for conflicting views
- investigate geographical variation
- identify Cinderella topics
- let loose the imagination

Review Existing Practice

Research ideas can come through reflection on current practice. It involves asking oneself a series of questions, to determine what happens to patients and what benefits they receive from their care. This review will help highlight topics for research. The types of questions which can help are:

- Why do we do it that way?
- If I were the patient what would I want?
- Do I really see all the patients that I could help?
- What do I do that is different to my colleagues?
- Where do things usually go wrong?
- When do I feel I'm wasting my time?
- Why did that patient not respond to the treatment?
- How could I have made the diagnosis more quickly?
- What other information would have improved management?
- Were all the investigations really necessary?
- What happens to these patients in the longer term?

The rationale behind these questions is that the current organisation and delivery of health care is not as good as it could be. The research questions focus either on identifying deficiencies or on developing better methods of delivery of care. A report on the recent initiative under the NHS Research and Development Strategy demonstrates just how many topics can be identified in this way. The report emphasises *'that there is indefensible diversity in the use of diagnostic methods and therapies and that there is unacceptable variation in the quality of treatment delivered by different clinical teams'* (7). In a separate initiative, an advisory group was set up to consider research priorities relating to the interface between primary and secondary care (8). In the course of four workshops over 200 issues were identified, which forced the group to prioritise them. They listed 10 top priorities (see Table 3.1), and 11 further priority areas. Although the interface between primary and secondary care may be a particularly fruitful area for research topics, this example illustrates the value of reflecting on current practice for identifying research topics.

Challenge Accepted Ideas

Much of health is based on accepted practice rather than research evidence, illustrated by the title of a recent BMJ editorial: *'Rituals in antenatal care—do we need them?'* (9). Many interventions are *'time honoured rather than proved'* (10). Sometimes practices become accepted because of enthusiastic advocacy rather than the weight of evidence. For example, the adoption of early intervention to accelerate labour, by rupturing membranes and prescribing oxytocin, has been traced to the *'vigorous prose style'* of a Dublin obstetrician (11). Although the old aphorism *'an accelerated labour is as safe as a streamlined parachute'* was

Table 3.1 Top priority topics at the interface between primary and secondary care

- Transfer of information across the interface between health care professionals and other agencies
- Evaluation of clinical guidelines at the interface
- Appropriate access, use and location of diagnostic facilities and new technologies
- Impact on referrals and discharge of involving patients and carers in decision making
- Appropriateness of out-patient follow-up
- Evaluation of treatment by referral versus management in primary care
- Impact of purchasing arrangements on the interface
- Aftercare: rehabilitation and community care for priority groups
- Prescribing across the interface
- Models of intermediate care

recalled, the practice spread into routine use, and only recently has sufficient evidence accumulated to challenge it (11).

Even practices which have official backing may be misplaced. For example, the size of a condom is specified by the British Standards Institute. But a research study found that some men *'have penises sufficiently large to cause difficulty in putting on condoms, and for those men condoms are likely to come off or split'* (12). In comparison with World Health Organization's guidelines, it appeared that over a third of British penises exceed the British Standards Institute's standard dimensions for condoms.

The point of these examples is to emphasise that research questions which challenge authority should not be abandoned. In contrast, it could be argued that one of the best places to look for research topics is among long-established practices: some may have been founded on misconceptions while others may have been overtaken by recent advances.

Look for Conflicting Views

Conflicting views on a topic, for example when some claim a treatment is effective and others disagree, indicate either that there is not enough evidence to decide the issue or that some practitioners are misinformed. In some instances it may not be clear whether conflict really exists, or if the extent of the conflict is sufficiently large to worry about. Rather than ignoring the issue it is possible to investigate it, to determine whether the conflict is real and, if so, to find out why. Thus one group, concerned about the management of neurogenic pain, surveyed the clinicians who treat this condition to ascertain their views on the available treatments (13, 14). They uncovered substantial disagreement about many treatments, identifying areas of educational need as well as confirming the existence of many topics requiring further research.

Conflicting views are often expressed at scientific meetings of medical societies, although people may be more willing to voice disagreement during the coffee break than in the lecture room. Another source is good review articles, which assess critically the current state of knowledge. Some journals also feature controversies among their articles. For example, the *British Medical Journal* began a series on controversy in management in the autumn of 1994, featuring such topics as the treatment of obesity (15), whether stroke patients are better managed in the community or in hospital (16), and the appropriateness of antibiotics for the treatment of sore throats (17). Areas of uncertainty identified in the literature can be picked out for further study.

Investigate Geographical Variation

There are widespread geographical variations in the frequency with which particular treatments are used. Reflection on the reasons these might occur can be a fruitful source of research questions. For example, consideration of the differing frequencies of prostatectomy for benign prostatic hyperplasia led to a number of research questions: What are the risks of a policy of watchful waiting? Which operation, transurethral resection or open surgery, has the lower long-term mortality? How is the success of the operation to be judged, urinary flow or patient symptoms? What do patients value more highly: relief of urinary dysfunction or preservation of sexual function? (18). All of these questions are potential topics for research.

Identify Cinderella Topics

Important areas of health care are often overlooked. For example, postoperative pain was largely ignored until comparatively recently. A report from the Royal College of Surgeons commented: *'the treatment of pain after surgery in British hospitals has been inadequate and has not advanced significantly for many years'* (19). Many patients experience severe pain which could be treated but is not. Fortunately, much research has been undertaken to document the extent of this problem and to uncover the reasons for patients suffering needless pain. This has enabled the Royal College of Surgeons to identify and recommend the changes in health care which are required to overcome the problem. It remains to be seen whether these measures are sufficient or whether further work is needed.

The areas of health care which are overlooked will include those in which research can contribute most to the improvement of patient care and well-being: *'if no one is investigating it there is probably a lot to be found out.'* This statement needs a little qualification, as some areas will be neglected deliberately because they are beyond the scope of present technology. However, many researchable topics will simply not have been considered, but remain unseen as pearls in unopened oysters. They can be identified by asking the types of questions listed under 'Reviewing existing practice', searching out those which have been relatively ignored.

Let Loose the Imagination

Finding a good research question is above all a matter of letting the imagination run free, to look for wild or impossible ideas. The intention is to free the mind from the constraints of conventional wisdom, to be able to challenge current practice. It does not matter that many of the ideas will be foolish: *'In the ordinary course of events scientists very often guess wrong, take a wrong view, or devise hypotheses that later turn out to be untenable'* (20). What is needed is a brainstorming approach to generate ideas without worrying whether they are sensible or foolish. At this first stage the usual critical faculty is suspended. Each aspect of current practice should be viewed from as many different angles as possible. Once the ideas have been identified they can then be assessed for their potential value and feasibility.

When ideas are being generated, it is essential they are not subject to critical assessment. New ideas may at first seem strange or unusual and they may contradict conventional wisdom. In a critical environment these ideas might never be voiced, lest they be deemed foolish. In truth, many of the ideas will be discarded, but it is only by going through the process that the potentially important areas will be identified.

STATING THE RESEARCH QUESTION

Having an idea for research is only the start of the process of developing the research question. Stating this question clearly and fully can be the most challenging part of research: *'the deceptively simple but dominating question, "what precisely am I trying to find out?"'* (21). The original idea could be thought of as a landscape which contains one or more good research questions, and many other features besides. This view clarifies that there are two stages in determining precisely what you are trying to find out:

* dissect out the research question(s)
* select the key question

Dissect out the Research Question(s)

When first expressed the research question may be vague or imprecise. This is not a problem, provided the question is subsequently clarified (see below). A common mistake when phrasing a research question is to recast the problem area as a general question of the form *'Why does this problem occur?'* This is quite unhelpful. Consider, for example, the problem of cervical cancer, a disease which should, in most cases, be preventable. A simple restatement of the problem would lead to the research question: *'Why do women continue to die from cervical cancer when effective screening could prevent this?'* This statement highlights an important public health issue, but as a research question it is quite useless. There are a large number of ways in which this issue could be approached, and the generally phrased question gives no indication of which one is to be followed. For example, the study could address the problem of non-usage of the service asking questions such as:

* What barriers deter some women from attending?
* What type of health promotion would encourage attendance?
* How could the service delivery be improved to encourage attendance?

Alternatively, interest could lie in determining whether women who have been screened develop cancer, asking questions such as:

* How accurately are smear results interpreted?
* How efficient is the follow-up of women with positive smears?
* What is the optimum interval between smears?

Or the study could look at the effectiveness of treatment, asking:

* How appropriate are the different forms of treatment (laser therapy, cone biopsy and hysterectomy)?
* Why do some women not attend for regular check-ups following treatment?

The cervical cancer example illustrates the large number of research questions which could be asked on this topic. What these questions have in common is that each focuses on a very limited part of the topic. Another feature of these questions is that they would involve collecting different types of data. It would be difficult and indeed foolish to try to answer them all in a single study. Most problem areas in health services research will, when inspected in detail, yield a variety of possible research questions. Only when the detailed questions have been teased out will feasible studies be able to be designed.

Strategies for Dissecting

Distilling the essence of a key question from a general research area is one of those activities which is easier to say than to do. However, a number of strategies can help:

- write out ideas
- discuss with colleagues
- think in the bath
- read around the subject
- look upstream

Write Out Ideas

When they first present, ideas can be tentative and vague, little more than an awareness that *'a research study could really help clarify this area'*. Sometimes these ideas are abandoned because they are far from being a coherent statement of a research project. Instead of losing them, it is a good practice to write them down. The process of writing may stimulate further ideas, and help clarify precisely what you want to do. Having the ideas on paper also means that you can add thoughts on how the study could be carried out and what value its findings might have. Findings from published reports can also be added as they are encountered, so that after germinating for some weeks or months, a prototype research project can be described.

Discuss with Colleagues

One of the easiest ways to clarify your own thoughts is to explain them to someone else. Being forced to put them into words means that the thoughts have to be organised in a logical structure so that the colleague may understand. This forces the mind to do something it tries to avoid:

to think deeply about the research idea. Even if the colleague has little comment to make, the episode will have been productive.

Think in the Bath

There is little doubt that ideas on research projects improve with age. They need to be mulled over, and allowed to mature: *'Really valuable research begins by thinking, not by doing. Banal questions produce banal answers'* (22). The varieties of research questions which could be asked will seldom be fully revealed at the first or even second episode of thinking. Instead, ideas often gradually develop and new questions suggest themselves on each occasion the topic is reviewed. To stimulate this type of thinking it can be helpful to ask oneself questions: What would I really like to do? What other ways could I approach this problem? What would be the easiest thing to find out? In a sense, this is having a conversation with oneself. It can bring additional benefits over discussions with colleagues because there is no need to explain the background to the research, and the conversation can follow illogical lines.

Read Around the Subject

Reading around the research area can help clarify thoughts on what might be done. It is important not just to read and think *'well, that is interesting'* (or alternatively that it is not). Reading should be an active process of asking questions about reported studies:

- Why did they do it?
- Why did they do it that way?
- Have any study details been omitted?
- Could I adapt their methods to my study?
- What scope is there for further research?
- Could the research methods be improved?

Often published papers conclude by suggesting further studies which need to be done, or even by stressing that their own study needs replication. For example, a report which appeared to show that vitamin supplementation improved the IQ of school children, ended with a request for a repeat study (23). When the replication was performed the effect was not confirmed (24).

However, there is a danger in reading: *'Too much book learning may crab and confine the imagination, and endless poring over the research of others is sometimes psychologically a research substitute, much as reading romantic fiction may be a substitute for real-life romance'* (25). The answer is to read selectively, skimming papers and taking advantage of review articles. The literature of any field is too vast for it all to be mastered. Instead, a self-critical approach can be adopted, asking after a visit to the library: Did I learn anything of real use? What were the most interesting papers? Could I have made better use of my time? Despite this caveat, reading the literature is an essential preliminary to research.

Look Upstream

The phrase look upstream refers to the metaphor of *'villagers who devised ever more complex technologies to save people from drowning, rather than looking up-river to see who was pushing them in'* (26). The analogy in health care is evident: for example, why try to develop a better drug for the control of diabetes if the current problem of management lies with patient compliance with existing effective therapies? Instead, research should be focused on the reasons for poor patient compliance and ways in which these can be overcome. Attention should concentrate on why events have occurred, seeking the origin of the causal chain.

Select the Key Question

The existence of a large number of possible questions, even within a single research area, and the need to focus on only one (or a small related set), raise the difficulty of how to decide which of the many to tackle. One approach is to rely on gut reaction to assess the value of the research question. This involves asking: Do I really want to find this out? Do I think that getting the answer is worth all the hassle? An enthusiastic *'yes'* suggests that there will be sufficient motivation to complete the study, and may indicate that an important question has been found.

An important question is not just one which gives more personal satisfaction when solved. There is undoubtedly an intellectual satisfaction of discovering new facts, and a professional pleasure in using these in practice. But, in an applied field like health services research, the real reward is in knowing that others have used your findings for the benefit of their patients.

Important problem areas are those in which new information is likely to bring about change, to lead to better delivery of health care. A good illustration of this is total hip replacement, which the Standing Group on Health Technology reviewed in their 1994 report (27). The reasons for concern about hip replacement were the variation in outcome, the uncertainty about which is the best type of prosthesis, and the increasing frequency of revision surgery. The report noted that both patients and the NHS would benefit from research which led to a reduced frequency of revision surgery. It was estimated that £26 million per year is currently being spent on revision surgery. The decision was easily taken that the potential benefits more than justified the costs of research, and research has been commissioned in this area.

The example of hip replacement illustrates some of the factors which can determine the potential value of a research question. In practice there are many such factors. The following list has been compiled and adapted from several sources (8, 27, 28):

- evidence for a problem
- burden of disease
- improvement of patient outcome
- cost implications
- likelihood of implementation
- need for early assessment
- feasibility of project

Evidence for the Problem

The starting point for assessment is the strength of the evidence that there really is a researchable question. The types of evidence which could be put forward include unexplained variations in the delivery of care, known variations in the outcome of care, evidence of unmet need, and conflict between published reports. All of these suggest that there is potential for research to improve the delivery of health care. They indicate that there may be a problem and lead to the next stage: assessing whether the problem is of sufficient magnitude to warrant investigation.

Burden of Disease

The burden of disease refers to the consequences for the individual and the community. A research question is likely to be important if it concerns a procedure or a disease which results in death. However, for many diseases, such as rheumatoid arthritis or migraine, death does not commonly happen. In these circumstances a disease would be considered important if it caused substantial disability or handicap, if it resulted in loss of quality of life. The term substantial reflects a balance between the size of effect for the individual and the number of individuals affected. For example, multiple sclerosis is not a common disease, but its effects on the individual can be devastating. In contrast, eczema-dermatitis is important because, although it has much less of an individual impact, it is much more common.

Improvement of Patient Outcome

Improvement of patient outcome is the inverse of the burden of illness. It could be assessed in terms of the prevention of death, decreased duration of illness, improved control of symptoms or increased quality of life. Again, importance is assessed as a balance between the size of the individual effect and the number of persons affected. Preventing even a few deaths is a major achievement. But just a small gain in the well-being of patients with a common disease like rheumatoid arthritis would be well worth having. Similarly, research which led to small improvements in the way common procedures are carried out would have substantial implications, making these topics worthwhile for study.

Cost Implications

Concern with costs is a characteristic of medicine in the 1990s. The greater the cost implications, such as the potential savings or the amount of avoidable waste, the greater the importance. Research can focus directly on economic issues, such as assessing the economic impact of chronic fatigue syndrome (29), or the costs and benefits of cardiac valve surgery (30). Cost can also be implicit in a study: for example, the finding by Dick and colleagues (31) of substantial inappropriate bed occupancy in an acute psychiatric ward has obvious financial implications even though these were not costed directly. Procedures like transplant surgery are inherently expensive, while diagnostic tests or screening procedures become expensive because of the frequency with which they are carried out. What is sometimes overlooked is that diseases or treatments can be important because of the length of time over which they last. Thus a prescription for anti-asthma medication may not be expensive, but as the condition is a chronic one the lifetime cost will be vast. The long-term prognosis is equally important for diseases like multiple sclerosis, a progressive degenerative disease. Although the condition is not common the total cost of treating this disabling illness is also large. In general, the greater the cost of a disease or procedure to the NHS, the more important it is likely to be as a topic for research.

Likelihood of Implementation

The recent focus on research and development within the NHS has highlighted the occurrence of delays between new discoveries being made, and these findings being adopted in practice: *'There are unacceptable delays in the implementation of many findings of research. This results in suboptimal care for patients'* (32). Delays can occur for a number of reasons. The implementation may require additional staff, or a higher grade of staff than currently in post. The new technique may be expensive. Some staff may be reluctant to adopt the innovation, preferring to *'wait and see how others find it'* (33). Whether this occurs will depend on the nature of the innovation, the possible hazards which it may carry and the strength of the entrenched view that it challenges. There may also be organisational barriers to implementation. Whatever the proposed area of research, these potential barriers need to be reviewed. If the barriers are thought to be insurmountable, the proposed research might have to be postponed or abandoned.

Need for Early Assessment

In some circumstances research can be of much more value if it is carried out immediately than if it is delayed for a few years. For example, when a new service, such as screening for breast cancer, is introduced there are clear advantages in evaluating its impact as early as possible. If it is shown to be ineffective, then early evaluation would lead more speedily to its cessation, with consequent savings. Further, once a new service becomes established, it becomes much more difficult to remove should it subsequently be shown to be ineffective. There may be substantial resistance from the staff employed in it and from the patients who use it. In general, timely research can both save more money and increase the likelihood that findings are implemented.

Feasibility of Project

The feasibility of a proposed study should be assessed at an early stage. Although the full study design need not be described, attention should be given to the questions: How do we do it? and Can we do it? If it is readily apparent that the study is not possible or that the design would be unethical, then it should be abandoned. Alternatively, anticipated technical problems can force a revision of the research question. The most common of these problems is the resources required to carry out the study. These include the number of staff and the types of expertise required and the equipment and materials which will be needed. If a project looks as though it might require more resources than are likely to be available, it should be put aside. Projects inevitably take more time and effort than expected.

REFINING THE QUESTION

Having identified a potentially worthwhile research question, attention needs to be given to refining it. Refining involves moulding and recasting until the question indicates precisely what the study intends to find out, and how it intends to do it. This position has been achieved when it is possible to state in some detail: the patient group to be studied; the data items to be collected; the features of the research method to be used; and the implications that the study findings could have for the delivery of health care. (Not that all of these details will be immutable: the study design will continue to evolve until data collection begins in earnest.)

Refining the question involves the same kinds of activities involved in finding the question in the first place: write ideas down, discuss with colleagues and think them over carefully. However, some additional advice may be helpful.

- review criteria of importance
- don't rush into a study
- review the analysis
- criticise
- be realistic

Review Criteria of Importance

The first step in refining a research question is to ask: How could the question be changed to make it more worthwhile? This will involve all the criteria which help identify important research questions (these were reviewed in the previous section). For example, one criterion of a good research question is the extent to which its findings will have wider implications. Thus a question could be refined by seeking out small changes which would increase its importance on this criterion. This is not a matter of stating the broad study area which is to be addressed, but of being specific about the ways in which the study findings could lead to improved patient care. Doing so will answer the questions: Why do we want to do this? Why is it worth doing? Where are the barriers to implementation? Who will be affected by the implementation? Answering these questions will help ensure that the research is worthwhile. They may force a revision to the research question, so that evidence is acquired to overcome the barriers to implementation. For example if the innovation has resource costs then it might be necessary to determine whether there might be potential savings as well. This refinement should identify those who may be affected by the findings, making it more likely that the study will be designed to provide results which will influence them.

Don't Rush into a Study

When a research question is first identified, the most important rule is not to rush into a study. In the first flush of enthusiasm there is a temptation to begin immediately. This should be resisted. The danger is of confusing action with progress, of doing rather than thinking. There are often many technical difficulties which can undermine a study. Thus it is best not to invest too much time and effort on any one aspect of a study, until it is reasonably certain that the whole study can be successfully carried out. For example, there is little point in developing a questionnaire to assess, say, the views of consultants on a specific therapy, until it is likely that the consultants can be contacted, and are willing to reply. Thus when refining the study question, first be sure it will work and be worthwhile.

Review the Analysis

Reviewing the analysis to be performed before the data are collected may seem a little premature, but it is an excellent practice. It helps to avoid the 'if only' syndrome. Many studies, as they near completion, are met with the groan: 'if only I had done it differently', as flaws in the basic design emerge during the analysis. One approach is to specify the tables which will be prepared, the graphs which will be drawn, and the statistical tests which will be used. The discipline of doing this focuses attention on the data to be collected, and specifically on the other factors that might influence the results. This will identify key variables which might not have been collected. It will also determine whether the question: What do I really want to find out? has been answered and whether the study design is sufficiently developed to enable the aims of the study to be met.

Criticise

In the initial stages of designing a research study attention is focused on the question: How can we make it succeed? At this time it is important not to be too critical, otherwise the weight of doubt and uncertainty will destroy the enthusiasm needed to develop the design. However, when the broad outline is decided and many of the detailed steps have been filled in comes the time for extensive criticism. Self-criticism can be difficult. The justified pride which a researcher may feel, having solved some of the major design problems, can leave more subtle but critical flaws overlooked. The researcher needs to play devil's advocate and look at the design like a jaundiced colleague. The questions now being asked are quite different to the earlier ones:

- where could it go wrong?
- why would people not participate?
- which data items might not be obtained?
- do we have sufficient resources and expertise?
- could a simpler method be used?

It is often helpful to put the design to one side for a few days, so that these questions can be looked at with a fresh eye. Another technique is to present the design to colleagues, perhaps as part of a research seminar, for discussion and comment. Only when the design has been tested in this fire of criticism can the study be commenced.

Be Realistic

All research studies contain imperfections: a few patients who cannot be traced, observer error in measurement, or known imperfections in available information (such as estimates of the costs of procedures). The important matter is not whether there might be flaws in a study, but whether these are sufficiently large as to invalidate the conclusions. The study does not need to be perfect, just good enough to answer the research question being posed. This realism helps ensure that important studies are not abandoned because of obvious but minor imperfections. This is not intended to encourage sloppiness; the study should be carried out as well as is practicable in the circumstances. Instead it is advising against an unattainable counsel of perfection.

REVIEWING PITFALLS

Research originates with an idea which is developed into a question. The question is clarified and refined, and its implications and feasibility are reassessed at every stage. There are many pitfalls for the unwary in the process of developing the research question. These have been alluded to in the preceding sections, but it is worth presenting the most common ones in a single place. These are:

- overelaborate and unfocused question
- insufficient commitment
- practicalities not assessed

The main pitfall of research design is to make a simple study difficult; to embroider the design with unwanted questions leading to the collection of unnecessary data. One of the main contributors to overelaborate studies consists in unfocused questions. Not specifying in detail the purposes of the study, the patient group to be studied or the measurements to be made often leads to the collection of large amounts of data. The only recourse is to clarify the details and to prune the less important questions.

The need for sufficient enthusiasm to complete a study is sometimes overlooked. If researchers are half-hearted about the enterprise and only doing it because they feel they must (through peer pressure or because promotion might depend on it), then the quality of the work will be poor. It is only when the researcher is genuinely interested in the research area, and wants to know the answer to the question posed, that the study may be completed to a high standard.

The role of planning has already been stressed in this chapter. Thinking through the possible methods and likely difficulties which might be encountered often leads to modifications to the research question. The remaining chapters of this book deal with the practicalities of the design, conduct, interpretation and dissemination of research studies. The next chapter begins this process by considering what can be learned from others through reviewing the published literature.

REFERENCES

1. Diamond, A. The future development of chronic pain relief [editorial]. *Anaesthesia* 1991; **46**: 83–4.
2. Melzack, R and Wall, PD. *The Challenge of Pain* 2nd edn. London: Penguin, 1988.

3. Budd, K. Recent advances in the treatment of chronic pain. *British Journal of Anaesthesia* 1989; **63**: 207–12.
4. Wells, JCD. The place of the pain clinic. *Baillières Clinical Rheumatology* 1987; **1**(1): 123–53.
5. Gaffney, G, Sellers, S, Flavell, V, Squier, M and Johnson, A. Case-control study of intrapartum care, cerebral palsy, and perinatal death. *British Medical Journal* 1994; **308**: 743–50.
6. Medawar, PB. *The Art of the Soluble*. Harmondsworth: Penguin, 1969: p169.
7. Peckham, M. Research and development for the National Health Service. *Lancet* 1991; **338**: 367–71.
8. Central Research and Development Committee Advisory Group. *R & D priorities in relation to the interface between primary and secondary care. Report to the NHS Central Research and Development Committee.* London: Department of Health, 1994.
9. Steer, P. Rituals in antenatal care—do we need them? [editorial]. *British Medical Journal* 1993; **307**: 697–8.
10. McQuay, H, Moore, A. Need for rigorous assessment of palliative care [editorial]. *British Medical Journal* 1994; **309**: 1315–16.
11. Thornton, JG and Lilford, RJ. Active management of labour: current knowledge and research issues. *British Medical Journal* 1994; **309**: 366–9.
12. Tovey, SJ and Bonell, CP. Condoms: a wider range needed. *British Medical Journal* 1993; **307**: 987.
13. Davies, HTO, Crombie, IK, Lonsdale, M and Macrae, WA. Consensus and contention in the treatment of chronic nerve-damage pain. *Pain* 1991; **47**: 191–6.
14. Davies, HTO, Crombie, IK and Macrae, WA. Polarised views on treating neurogenic pain. *Pain* 1993; **54**: 341–6.
15. Garrow, JS. Should obesity be treated? Treatment is necessary. *British Medical Journal* 1994; **309**: 654–5.
16. Young, J. Is stroke better managed in the community? Community care allows patients to reach their full potential. *British Medical Journal* 1994; **309**: 1356–7.
17. Little, PS and Williamson, I. Are antibiotics appropriate for sore throats? Costs outweigh the benefits. *British Medical Journal* 1994; **309**: 1010–11.
18. Delamothe, T. Using outcomes research in clinical practice [editorial]. *British Medical Journal* 1994; **308**: 1583–4.
19. Working Party of the Royal College of Surgeons of England and the College of Anaesthetists. *Pain after Surgery*. London: Commission on the Provision of Surgical Services, 1990.
20. Medawar, P. *The Threat and the Glory: Reflections on Science and Scientists.* Oxford: Oxford University Press, 1991: p73.
21. Hill, AB. Heberden Oration, 1965. Reflections on the controlled trial. *Annals of Rheumatic Diseases* 1966; **25**: 107–13.
22. McCormick, J. Eschewing the predictable. *Lancet* 1994; **344**: 1243–4.
23. Benton, D and Roberts, G. Effect of vitamin and mineral supplementation on intelligence of a sample of schoolchildren. *Lancet* 1988; **i**: 140–3.
24. Crombie, IK, Todman, J, McNeill, G, Florey, CdV, Menzies, I and Kennedy, RA. Effect of vitamin and mineral supplementation on verbal and non-verbal reasoning of schoolchildren. *Lancet* 1990; **335**: 744–7.
25. Medawar, PB. *Advice to a Young Scientist*. New York: Harper & Row, 1979: 16.

26. Population health looking upstream [editorial]. *Lancet* 1994; **343**: 429–30.
27. Standing Group on Health Technology. *1994 Report*. London: Department of Health, 1994.
28. Crombie, IK, Davies, HTO, Abraham, SCS and Florey, CdV. *The Audit Handbook: Improving Health Care through Clinical Audit*. Chichester: John Wiley & Sons, 1993.
29. Lloyd, AR, Pender H. The economic impact of chronic fatigue syndrome. *Medical Journal of Australia* 1992; **157**: 599–601.
30. Thick, MG, Lewis, CT, Weaver, EJM and Flavell, G. An attempt to measure the costs and benefits of cardiac valve surgery at the London Hospital in adults of working age. *Health Trends* 1978; **10**: 58–60.
31. Dick, PH, Crombie, IK, Durham, T, McFee, C, Primrose, M and Mitchell, S. Unnecessary hospitalisation in a psychiatric rehabilitation unit. *British Medical Journal* 1992; **304**: 1544.
32. Haines, A and Jones, R. Implementing findings of research. *British Medical Journal* 1994; **308**: 1488–92.
33. Clinical trials and clinical practice [editorial]. *Lancet* 1993; **342**: 877–8.

Chapter 4

REVIEWING THE LITERATURE

Reviewing the literature is an essential activity for several stages of a research project. A review of published work will show which areas have already been tackled and the success achieved. It will identify the methods which could be used, and give some indication of the problems which might be encountered. It may reveal inconsistencies in findings between studies which could indicate areas for further research. Finally, many papers contain suggestions for further investigation. This chapter describes how a literature search may be carried out, and then reviews the critical assessment of published papers.

CONDUCTING THE SEARCH

There are usually a number of specialist libraries in large towns and cities: hospitals, medical schools, nursing colleges, dental colleges will all have separate libraries. They differ in the types of books and journals they contain; for example, the psychiatric hospital libraries have fewer general medical journals, but more on mental illness and suicide. Thus an important question to ask before beginning a literature search is: Which library should be used? Sometimes the answer may be more than one, to take advantage of the specialised collections which each may hold.

Another question which can usefully be asked before entering the library is: Can I get advice from colleagues before beginning? Someone locally may have an interest in a similar area, and may already have compiled a list of references. Or they may know of key researchers in the field to whom you can write. It is quite acceptable to write to someone you do not know and ask for copies of papers they have published; most researchers are pleased when others take an interest in their work.

The literature search itself involves several different activities:

- planning the search
- getting started

- being selective
- filing
- stopping

Planning the Search

Libraries are full of interesting papers and books, and many happy hours can be passed browsing. To ensure time is used to best advantage a number of decisions need to be made before beginning the search, including:

- the breadth of the search
- the depth of the search
- the period of the search

Before starting some thought needs to be given to the particular purposes of the search. Is it just a toe-dip to get a feel for what is going on, or is it to obtain detailed information on a specific subject? When investigating a new topic the first search is often brief; it may be sufficient to rely on a recent book or a few review articles. Detailed searches can pose problems. Suppose the research addressed the management of childhood asthma. The researcher might want to know how common the condition is in children, how serious it is, what treatments are available, and what guidance is given on management. As well as studies on asthma in children, it could be useful to look at the literature on asthma in adults. This would include studies on the effectiveness of the differing treatments (many more studies on effectiveness are carried out on adults than on children). The reasons for the disease being poorly managed could also be investigated. Is it lack of recognition of the problem by the GP, or because of poor compliance by the children? The literature search would need to be extended to include these areas. Further, as asthma is a chronic condition, it could be useful to review its natural history. Thus before entering the library the researcher should have compiled a list of subjects including: asthma frequency, severity and natural history; effectiveness of treatments; diagnosis of asthma; and factors affecting patient compliance.

The way the search is approached also needs to be considered carefully. The literature is often approached with a specific disease in mind, but there may be benefit in searching for processes and procedures in other areas. For example if the interest is in patient compliance with therapy, key papers on the topic could be published in psychology journals without reference to a specific disease. Similarly, papers on service delivery in rheumatology (e.g. shared care schemes) could have relevance for the organisation of services in chest clinics. The search may need to be cast wider than the specific disease.

The number of years of literature to be searched will also have to be decided. When searching for review articles it might be sufficient to concentrate on the recent past, but a longer period may be needed for original papers. There are no hard and fast rules for the period of the search, except to say that it would seem unwise to restrict the search to recent years. The decision will depend on how novel the topic is, and how likely it is that important papers might have been published seven or eight years ago. If the field is one of intensive study there might be too many papers to read if more than a few years are reviewed. In this instance it would be better to rely on review articles to identify the older papers and to concentrate the search on the more recent ones.

One final word on planning: expect to be disappointed. Often the key paper which you want will not exist. The feeling that *'surely someone has made a clear statement on this issue'* will often be met with the finding that no one has. Careful inspection may reveal a few nuggets cast away as asides in some papers, but in other instances the search may be fruitless. One area in which information will often be lacking is the methodological and logistical problems of conducting studies. Medical journals are heavily focused on findings. Information will often be sparse on the workload involved in a study, the resources required, and the potential pitfalls in study conduct.

Getting Started

The first foray into the library to start reviewing the literature is undoubtedly the most difficult. It is not always easy to identify the key papers, recent books or review articles. The difficulties are compounded if there has been insufficient planning and the researcher is unclear what is wanted. A good starting point is to ask a colleague or a local professional with an interest in the area for some advice. But local professionals tend to be too busy to give more than limited advice. There is no alternative to searching for yourself. Fortunately, libraries have a number of facilities to simplify the literature review:

- indexing journals
- computerised searches
- review articles
- bibliographies/abstracting journals

The people who know most about these facilities are the local library staff, and it is essential to make friends with them. They understand how books and journals are indexed and stored, and can give advice on how to do a literature search, find missing books and articles, order books or journals not held locally, or recall books lent to other readers. Like all professionals, librarians usually enjoy explaining their subject to others, so never be afraid to ask for help.

Indexing Journals

There are some specialised journals, such as *Index Medicus, Excerpta Medica*, and the *Science and Social Science Citation Indices*, which list details of papers published in professional journals. Their use can be illustrated by focusing on one, *Index Medicus*, as all three are organised in broadly the same way. *Index Medicus* covers over 2700 biomedical journals worldwide. It is issued monthly throughout the year, but it is easier to use the annual cumulative editions, unless you really need to be right up to date. *Index Medicus* lists articles by subject and by author, and it also lists review articles separately. Each listing gives the title of the paper and its publication details, so that the original article can be located.

The first step in using *Index Medicus* is to draw up a list of the key terms on which you wish to search. These are referred to as MeSH headings (**Me**dical **S**ubject **H**eadings). Asthma is a MeSH heading, and within it papers are arranged in a series of subcategories such as diagnosis, drug therapy, etiology, prevention and control, and therapy. It is an American publication and thus uses American spelling and terminology, which can cause confusion. For example, there is no entry for cancer: the MeSH heading is neoplasm.

Great care must be taken in choosing MeSH headings. Papers may not be listed under the heading which seems most obvious to the researcher. Thus searches would need to be carried out using several different headings to ensure that all relevant papers are found. For example, if the topic were asthma treatment, searching under the specific treatments such as bronchodilators (another MeSH heading) could yield additional papers.

Computerised Searches

Manual searches through *Index Medicus* can be very time consuming. Fortunately, it has been computerised and many libraries have up to date copies on CD-ROM, a conventional compact disc which can be read by a computer (this is just a convenient method of storing large amounts of information). It is accessed in the same way, through MeSH headings, although some help may be needed from the librarian to use the computer. For many of the papers indexed a copy of the abstract is also available, making it much easier to decide which papers are relevant. An additional benefit of the computerised system is that the selected references can be printed out, obviating the need for tedious manual copying. Information may also be written to a floppy disc and taken away for later inspection.

One useful feature is the facility to select only those articles where MeSH headings represent a substantial part of the contents. The headings also have assigned subheadings which can be used to narrow down the search. The subheadings available depend on the particular heading which has been chosen, but frequently available ones include Diagnosis, Aetiology, Surgery and Drug Therapy.

The same degree of care needs to be taken in specifying the MeSH headings for computerised searches as with the manual method, and several related headings should be used. The computerised system not only makes it possible to carry out repeated searches in a few seconds, but it allows searches to be carried out using combinations of headings. This can be useful because searches on many MeSH headings will often identify hundreds if not thousands of references. By selecting combinations of headings, the search can be greatly narrowed.

Searches can also be conducted based on words appearing in the title or abstract. For example, if neoplasm is the selected word, all papers in which this word appears in the title or abstract can be identified. However, there is a drawback: there must be an exact match between the textword specified and the one appearing in the paper. Different forms of the same word will not be recognised. For example, if neoplasm were specified then neoplastic and neoplasia would not be recognised. One solution to this is to truncate the term to say 'neopla', and tell the computer that this is a truncated word (by adding a $ sign as a suffix). Then all words which contain the root 'neopla' will be recognised. Another difficulty of using textwords as the basis for a search is spelling differences between American and English words: gynecology and gynaecology; paediatrics and pediatrics. Searches would have to use both forms of these words to cover journals published in both countries.

Computerised searches are very simple to undertake, but they need to be carefully planned. They have limitations. Studies which have compared extensive manual searches with computerised searches find that the computer will provide somewhere between 50% and 90% of the papers which the manual search would uncover (1, 2). If the topic is an important one there may be no alternative but to search through selected journals, especially those not covered by *Index Medicus*.

The ease with which many tens of thousands of papers can be scanned in a computer search can lead to further problems. Large numbers of potentially relevant papers may be identified. The search can be narrowed by using combinations of MeSH headings and textwords, but even then there may be more than 100 references to be inspected. The only recourse is to scan them quickly, ruthlessly discarding those which may only be of peripheral interest. There is not enough time to read them all.

Citation Indices

The *Science and Social Science Citation Indices* have one feature that the other indexing journals do not: they allow you to track a paper forwards through time. Suppose you have identified one of the landmark studies in a particular field. Subsequent studies in the same field are almost certain to cite this paper. These more recent studies could be identified if there were a list of the papers which cited the landmark study. This is what the *Science and Social Science Citation Indices* provide. For all the papers published in a calendar year, they list the references which these papers have cited. The list is arranged by the surname of the first author of the cited papers, and gives details of all the papers which cited it. Not all of the studies which are identified will be relevant, but some will. Cynics may claim that the principal use of the tracking facility is for researchers to check whether anyone has cited their own published work. Whatever the truth of that claim, these citation indices are a powerful tool in literature searches.

Review Articles

Review articles can provide a simple means of entry to the research literature. Most journals publish occasional reviews, and there are many journals dedicated to expert reviews covering a wide range of topics. For example, the *British Medical Bulletin* (published by Churchill Livingstone) has recently reviewed alcohol problems, assisted human conception, hearing and perioperative care. Another excellent source of reviews are the *Effective Health Care* bulletins (published by the School of Public Health, University of Leeds) with recent titles including screening for osteoporosis and stroke rehabilitation. *Index Medicus* also compiles a list of review articles from the journals included in its search. There are too many of these types of journals for them all to be listed here, but it would be easy to check which are available locally.

Bibliographies/Abstracting Journals

There are several publications which provide lists of references. For example, *Current Bibliographies in Medicine* (National Library of Medicine, USA) does so for selected topics covering papers over the previous few years. In contrast, *Current Contents in Medicine* (produced by the Institute for Scientific Information) gives a weekly listing of references to the papers published in some 900 journals. Other journals, for example the *Health Service Abstracts* (published by the Department of Health), provide summaries of the papers as well as the details of the reference. If any of these are available locally they can be a useful source of references.

Being Selective

There are many more published papers which might be relevant to a research study than a researcher could possibly read. Instead, papers need to be read selectively and progressively. A quick skim through the abstract should indicate whether the paper is worth more detailed review, asking: Will this provide me with information that I need? Only if the answer is a definite *'yes'* should it be read further; if the answer is *'well, it might be useful sometime'* then it should be filed.

Filing

Filing is a somewhat dull word for a very important activity. Having made the effort to collect a set of references, they need to be organised so that they can be retrieved easily. It is a good practice to photocopy key papers, so that they are always to hand. Photocopied papers quickly accumulate into disorganised piles, making it difficult to find that key study when it is needed. If a paper can't be found when it is wanted, there is little point in having it. Obviously the papers need to be filed. But when entering a new area it can be difficult to decide which categories to allocate papers to. The answer is to have a stab at it (dividing them up by type of study, purpose of study, type of patients, etc.), without worrying too much whether the system works properly. When there are only a few papers, it will still be relatively easy to find particular studies. Then when the numbers in any category increase and the system begins to look heterogeneous, it can be subdivided. The process of gradually subdividing categories will lead towards a more sensible classification system.

Some papers may be relevant to more than one of the filing categories, and it can be difficult to decide which one to choose. It would be wasteful to make two copies, but filing in one place might lead to an important paper being overlooked. A compromise would be to photo-copy the front page of the paper, cross-referencing it to the location of the complete article. For those who have their own computers, an alternative would be to use a bibliographic database. This is a computer program which stores details of the reference, the category in which it is filed, and any key words that the researcher wishes to add. The reference can be called up by either the author's name, any word in the title, or any of the keywords which have been entered. Thus papers can be found easily by searching your own literature collection. Perhaps the greatest benefit of a computerised database is the way it simplifies the task of compiling lists of references for papers and reports.

Finally, all this talk of filing should not divert attention from the important task of reading the papers themselves. Filing is not an end in itself. There is little point in having a beautiful filing system if the material in it is never used.

Stopping

Dangers lurk in all forms of exploration and literature searches are no exception. Many papers cite interesting references, and when these are chased up they mention other interesting papers. Many hours can be spent collecting and reading the resulting papers. Although an enjoyable activity, extensive reading can easily consume the little time that a health professional has for research. Unless you are writing the ultimate authoritative review, there is no need to cover all the papers in an attempt to be comprehensive. Instead, if the purpose of the search has been clearly established, then the searching can be stopped when that purpose has been fulfilled. In many instances there will be several studies which draw the same broad conclusions: for example postoperative pain is poorly managed; or asthma is under-recognised. Having established what is going on, the search can be terminated.

READING THE LITERATURE

Papers may be read in different ways. Not all need to be reviewed in detail. Some will be read in depth because their methods or their findings bear directly on your own study, while for others a quick skim may be sufficient. To help decide the depth to which a book, paper or report should be read it is helpful to preview it, to inspect it before reading it in more detail. The preview can involve looking briefly at the headings and subheadings, the abstract or parts of the discussion, or the tables and figures. Previewing provides an overview, a framework, within which further information from the paper can be organised. It will also determine whether the paper needs to be read in detail, because the results may be interesting or because other parts of the paper contain useful information. There are two types of question which may be asked when approaching a paper, and it is useful to consider them separately.

- what lessons can be learned?
- what do the findings mean?

Lessons to be Learned

Different types of information can be obtained from the various parts of the paper. The Introduction and Discussion sections may provide new references, present novel ways of thinking about health care problems, or even suggest areas for further research. The Methods section may describe useful ways of making measurements or identifying patients for study. This section may also describe pitfalls that were encountered, or give details of statistical methods that can be used. The Results section is the one which usually shows how things can go wrong: the amount of missing data; the unusual nature of the study group; the inconsistencies in the results. Learning from the experiences of others is one way of improving the quality of one's own research.

The basis of the lesson learning approach is that even papers which are fatally flawed can contain useful information. For example, the results of a study may have little value because data could not be obtained on key groups of patients. The lesson is that future studies would have to be carried out in a quite different way to ensure that valid results are obtained.

Interpreting the Findings

Critical inspection of published studies often finds them to be deficient. One review of health services research reported that *'major inadequacies were found in the conduct of research, particularly in the selection of controls, allowance for confounding factors, objectivity of measurements, application of statistical tests, and conclusions reached'* (3). Several surveys of published papers have found that *'about half the articles that used statistical methods did so incorrectly'* (4–6). A recent book has collected a substantial series of studies with methodological errors (7). Reading these is an excellent way to hone critical skills.

In the critical assessment of papers the overriding question is: Am I persuaded by this study's results? Answering this involves asking a series of other questions:

- How was it done?
- Why was it done that way?
- How could it have been done better?
- What do the results actually mean?
- What other explanations could there be for the findings?
- Are there flaws or biases which could invalidate the findings?

Asking these questions will inevitably reveal flaws in many papers, but they should not necessarily be discarded. It is always possible to find a potential bias, or statistical quibble. Few studies are perfect. But small deficiencies in design or analysis may not matter. The question is not whether there are flaws or biases, but whether any of these could have a large enough effect to vitiate the conclusions from the study.

The above questions are general ones, and there are a second set of more detailed ones which could be asked (see Table 4.1). These have been developed from a number of papers which provide checklists for critically assessing papers and guidance on how to detect statistical errors (4, 8–11). Not all the questions will be appropriate for each type of study, although it should be evident from the context which will be relevant. The basic approach is to ask each question in turn and then decide if there is a potential problem, and whether it is large enough to be of concern.

Critical assessment of the literature is a skill which takes practice to develop. It is a much wider topic than can be covered here. Those wishing to read more about it will benefit from the series of papers in the *Canadian Medical Association Journal* (12–16) and the *Journal of the American Medical Association* (17–23). There is also a good book by

Table 4.1 Checklist for the critical assessment of papers

Study group
Was the source of subjects clearly defined?
Is the study group likely to be representative of a wider group?
Were exclusion and inclusion criteria defined?
Was the method of sampling described? (e.g. consecutive subjects, or randomly selected subjects)

Control groups
Was one used? If not should one have been used?
If a control group was used:
Was it appropriate, or likely to differ systematically from the study group?
Were data collected in the same way as for the study group?

Study design
Is the design appropriate to the stated objectives?
Was the period of observation/treatment sufficiently long to detect an effect?
If used, was the treatment adequately described and clinically appropriate?

Study conduct
Were all the subjects considered for entry to the study accounted for?
Was information given on non-responders, non-compliance, drop-outs or other sources of missing data?

Measurements
Were the circumstances and methods of measurement fully described?
Are the measurements likely to be valid and reliable?
Were the measurements which were made the most clinically relevant given the study aims?
Were some relevant outcomes omitted?
Was observation blinded where relevant?

Analysis
Were the statistical methods described and if so were they appropriate for the data?
Are the assumptions underlying the statistical methods likely to be met?
Was allowance made for confounding factors?

Interpretation
Were the conclusions justified?
Were the limitations of the study acknowledged and taken into account ?
Were alternative explanations considered?
Is an overemphasis given to positive findings with negative findings being dismissed?
Was the study sufficiently large to be likely to detect clinically important findings?
Was the clinical significance of the findings commented on?

Gehlbach (24) on reading the literature. Those with a substantial literature to cover may benefit by learning some of the techniques to improve speed and comprehension of reading (25).

COMMENT AND FURTHER READING

This chapter has outlined the approaches which can be taken to identify relevant papers in the medical literature. The process begins with a careful appraisal of what is really being sought and the depth to which the search should be conducted. There are a number of useful facilities to assist in the search, including indexing journals, computerised searches, and bibliographic/abstracting journals.

The number of potentially relevant papers is vast, so that they must be collected selectively. If a first attempt at searching turns out to be insufficient, further searches can always be undertaken. The papers collected need to be organised so that each can be retrieved when it is wanted. The papers themselves need to be read critically, as many may contain major flaws or errors which negate their conclusions. However, papers should not be rejected because of minor deficiencies, but instead the reader should ask: What can I usefully learn from this paper?

This chapter can only provide a brief coverage of methods of reviewing the literature. Advice on how to use a medical library is given in a book by Morton and Wright (26). Two other books describe how to search and interpret the medical literature (27, 28). More details on how to use *Index Medicus* and *Excerpta Medica* are given in a second book by Strickland-Hodge (29). A worldwide listing of indexing journals, online databases, bibliographies, symposia and conference series is given by Kurian (30). But the best advice is to ask your local librarian.

REFERENCES

1. Chalmers, I, Dickersin, K and Chalmers, TC. Getting to grips with Archie Cochrane's agenda [editorial]. *British Medical Journal* 1992; **305**: 786–8.
2. Smith, BJ, Darzins, PJ, Quinn, M and Heller, RF. Modern methods of searching the medical literature. *Medical Journal of Australia* 1992; **157**: 603–11.
3. Fowkes, FGR, Garraway, WM and Sheehy, CK. The quality of health services research in medical practice in the United Kingdom. *Journal of Epidemiology and Community Health* 1991; **45**: 102–6.
4. Glantz, SA. Biostatistics: how to detect, correct and prevent errors in the medical literature. *Circulation* 1980; **61**(1): 1–7.

5. Lionel, NDW and Herxheimer, A. Assessing reports of therapeutic trials. *British Medical Journal* 1970; **3**: 637–40.
6. Gore, SM, Jones, IG and Rytter, EC. Misuse of statistical methods: critical assessment of articles in BMJ from January to March 1976. *British Medical Journal* 1977; **1**: 85–7.
7. Andersen, B. *Methodological Errors in Medical Research*. Oxford: Blackwell Scientific Publications, 1990.
8. Gore, SM, Jones, G and Thompson, SG. The *Lancet*'s statistical review process: areas for improvement by authors. *Lancet* 1992; **340**: 100–2.
9. Gardner, MJ, Machin, D and Campbell, MJ. Use of check lists in assessing the statistical content of medical studies. *British Medical Journal* 1986; **292**: 810–12.
10. Fowkes, FGR and Fulton, PM. Critical appraisal of published research: introductory guidelines. *British Medical Journal* 1991; **302**: 1136–40.
11. Altman, DG, Gore, SM, Gardner, MJ and Pocock, SJ. Statistical guidelines for contributors to medical journals. *British Medical Journal* 1983; **286**: 1489–93.
12. Department of Clinical Epidemiology and Biostatistics MUHSC. How to read clinical journals: I. Why to read them and how to start reading them critically. *Canadian Medical Association Journal* 1981; **124**: 555–8.
13. Department of Clinical Epidemiology and Biostatistics MUHSC. How to read clinical journals: II. To learn about a diagnostic test. *Canadian Medical Association Journal* 1981; **124**: 703–10.
14. Department of Clinical Epidemiology and Biostatistics MUHSC. How to read clinical journals: III. To learn the clinical course and prognosis of disease. *Canadian Medical Association Journal* 1981; **124**: 869–72.
15. Department of Clinical Epidemiology and Biostatistics MUHSC. How to read clinical journals: IV. To determine etiology or causation. *Canadian Medical Association Journal* 1981; **124**: 985–90.
16. Department of Clinical Epidemiology and Biostatistics MUHSC. How to read clinical journals: V. To distinguish useful from useless or even harmful therapy. *Canadian Medical Association Journal* 1981; **124**: 1156–62.
17. Oxman, AD, Sackett, DL and Guyatt, GH. Users' guides to the medical literature. I. How to get started. *Journal of the American Medical Association* 1993; **270**(17): 2093–5.
18. Guyatt, GH, Sackett, DL and Cook, DJ. Users' guides to the medical literature. II. How to use an article about therapy or prevention. A. Are the results of the study valid? *Journal of the American Medical Association* 1993; **270**(21): 2598–601.
19. Guyatt, GH, Sackett, DL and Cook, DJ. Users' guides to the medical literature. II. How to use an article about therapy or prevention. B. What were the results and will they help me in caring for my patients? *Journal of the American Medical Association* 1994; **271**(1): 59–63.
20. Jaeschke, R, Guyatt, G and Sackett, DL. Users' guides to the medical literature. III. How to use an article about a diagnostic test. A. Are the results of the study valid? *Journal of the American Medical Association* 1994; **271**(5): 389–91.
21. Jaeschke, R, Guyatt, GH and Sackett, DL. Users' guides to the medical literature. III. How to use an article about a diagnostic test. B. What are the results and will they help me in caring for my patients? *Journal of the American Medical Association* 1994; **271**(9): 703–7.

22. Laupacis, A, Wells, G, Richardson, WS, Tugwell, P. Users' guides to the medical literature. V. How to use an article about prognosis. *Journal of the American Medical Association* 1994; **272**(3): 234–7.

23. Levine, M, Walter, S, Lee, H, Haines, T, Holbrook, A and Moyer, V. Users' guides to the medical literature. IV. How to use an article about harm. *Journal of the American Medical Association* 1994; **271**(20): 1615–19.

24. Gehlbach, SH. *Interpreting the Medical Literature* 3rd edn. New York: McGraw-Hill, 1993.

25. Buzan, T. *Speed Reading*. London: Guild Publishing, 1988.

26. Morton, LT and Wright, DJ. *How to Use a Medical Library* 7th edn. London: Library Association Publishing, 1990.

27. Livesey, B and Strickland-Hodge, B. *How to Search the Medical Sources*. Aldershot: Gower, 1989.

28. Warren, KS, ed. *Coping with the Biomedical Literature: A Primer for the Scientist and the Clinician*. New York: Praeger, 1981.

29. Strickland-Hodge, B. *How to use Index Medicus and Excerpta Medica*. Aldershot: Gower, 1986.

30. Kurian, GT. *Global Guide to Medical Information*. New York: Elsevier, 1988.

Chapter 5

CASE REPORTS AND CASE SERIES

The study of new or interesting cases has played a central role in medicine. This can involve the detailed investigation of one or a few cases, or the more systematic collection of information on a larger series. This chapter reviews both approaches, outlining their uses, their strengths, and the weaknesses that they are heir to.

CASE REPORTS

Case reports typically derive from astute clinical observation, when an unusual case is identified and its significance realised. They have a range of uses.

Uses

Case reports describe the presenting signs and symptoms of a disease, its progress, or its response to treatment. They can contribute to the identification of:

- new diseases
- adverse outcomes of treatment
- causes of rare diseases

Clusters of cases with similar but unusual symptoms can lead to the identification of new diseases. The identification of AIDS followed the occurrence of a few cases of rare pneumonias and Karposi's sarcoma among homosexual men in Los Angeles. New diseases seldom pose such a worldwide threat, but they can be clinically important. For example, an investigation was conducted into an outbreak of an un-diagnosed severe respiratory disease in the southwestern United States. The clinical course was of rapid progressive acute pulmonary oedema, with a case-fatality rate of 76%. But the cause of the disease proved difficult to identify: *'laboratory tests for bacterial and viral pathogens and a variety of toxic agents were negative'* (1). Further laboratory work identified a new strain of hantavirus as the cause of disease.

Case reports are often the means by which adverse reactions to drugs are first identified. For example, adenosarcoma of the vagina is extremely rare in young women, so the observation of seven cases diagnosed over a short interval gave rise to concern (2). Further investigation showed that it was diethylstilboestrol taken by mothers during pregnancy which led to this cancer in their daughters.

Case reports are not limited to identifying problems associated with the use of drugs, they can also identify unexpected outcomes following surgery. The efficacy of vasectomy was called into question by the collection of six cases of men who fathered children after they had had this operation (3). All the men produced persistently negative semen samples, but DNA analysis showed that they were the fathers. The authors of the report concluded that patients *'should be warned of the small possibility of late failure of the operation'*.

Case reports can suggest new causes of existing disease. Thus silicone implants for breast augmentation have been linked to the sporadic occurrence of scleroderma. However, this type of evidence cannot confirm a causal relationship, it can only indicate where further research, using formal research methods, is warranted (see Chapters 6–9). Further research on silicone implants showed they carry no risk (4).

Advantages

Case reports are simple to carry out, involving little more than the review of clinical material. One of their strengths is their ability to disprove accepted hypotheses: only one black swan is required to refute the statement that all swans are white. Thus the occurrence of a single case of smallpox, a disease which was eradicated in the 1970s, would be sufficient to show that there was a new source of the disease.

Weaknesses

Case reports commonly focus on cases which are unusual, with the unstated hope that this unusualness will lead to unexpected findings. However, if the case is unique or at best extremely rare, then the finding may have little practical importance. Further, the process of selecting cases may result in such a set of atypical patients that the results are positively misleading. Case reports should always be considered to be *'preliminary observations and highly subject to subsequent refutation . . . [they] do not permit discrimination of the valid from the interesting but erroneous'* (5).

One area in which case reports are singularly unhelpful is in the evaluation of the efficacy of treatments. There are several instances where case reports have suggested that a new treatment was effective which large and more rigorous studies subsequently show to be of no value or even harmful. For example gastric freezing seemed a possible treatment for peptic ulcer, because it had been found that cooling the stomach, by introducing coolant into a gastric balloon, substantially reduced acid secretion. The first few patients who were treated appeared to benefit greatly, with the result that gastric freezing machines were widely used. Only when a large study compared the outcomes in treated and untreated patients was the treatment shown to be ineffective (6). In general a few enthusiastic reports, particularly when coming from the clinicians who pioneered the new treatment, should not be used as the basis for changing medical practice.

In summary, case reports may provide useful information: they can indicate that previously held views may be suspect; and can identify instances where care was deficient. However, they are not a method for answering research questions.

EXTENDING CASE REPORTS: CASE SERIES

The obvious extension to the case report is the systematic collection of data on a large number of cases: *'the age-old cornerstone of medical progress, the case series'* (7). This would appear to overcome the potential pitfall of unusualness which besets case reports. Case series have contributed to knowledge in a number of ways, including the assessment of the safety of procedures or treatments. A classical example of this type of use are the two series collected by John Snow in 1847 which *'helped to dispel the mistrust of ether anaesthesia which had been engendered by inept applications in England in 1846'* (8).

Dangers

Case series can be relatively easy to carry out. Data can be collected on patients as they are seen, or abstracted subsequently from casenotes.

Because of their relative simplicity, case series might appear an attractive approach to research: *'few things come more intuitively to a practising physician than to collect information on patients with a certain disease to see whether these people have something strange in common'* (7). They might be used to ask a number of questions: What are the patients like? How well were they managed? How does their disease progress? How well do they respond to treatment? What further treatments are they given? However, the simplicity of the approach is deceptive, and as a research method the case series has serious weaknesses.

Perhaps the gravest danger of collecting a series of cases is that it is done because it appears straightforward rather than to answer a particular research question. It is often of little value to ask: *'What are my patients like?'* The answer will usually be *'much like anyone else's'* and be of little interest to anyone. Equally, there is little point in collecting lots of data in the hope that some interesting results will pop out: magicians may pull rabbits out of hats, but in research new findings seldom leap out from data collected without purpose. The cardinal rule is do not begin data collection unless there is a good reason for it, a focused well-defined question to be answered. There are countless filing cabinets throughout the world filled with case series that will never see the light of day. Sadly the effort of collecting cases simply uses the time and energy which could have been spent completing other research studies. (This is not an invitation to discard records wilfully, as old records can sometimes prove useful. Instead, it is a caution against wasting time collecting information without having a good purpose for doing so.)

Differing Guises

Often the case series is really another method in disguise, commonly a survey. An example of this is the report by Neale (9) on legal claims against hospital doctors. It presented a review of 100 successive cases submitted by solicitors to a consultant physician for a medical opinion. Although in 44 cases no serious clinical errors had occurred, 13 of the cases were major errors due to carelessness or incompetence. The problem with these estimates is that they depend on the way that solicitors chose to send cases to the physician. It is possible that the consultant was a highly respected figure to whom only the most complex cases were sent. The report acknowledged that the cases sent reflected the doctor's special interest in gastroenterology and general medicine. Thus the cases that were reviewed could well be different from the general run of medicolegal cases, i.e. the cases might not be representative. It is the possibility of lack of representativeness that makes case series an uncertain method for research. In some instances useful information can be obtained from case series, but on other occasions the results can be misleading. It would be better to acknowledge from the outset that a survey was being conducted, and then to review the limitations and pitfalls to which surveys are prone (see Chapter 6 for details).

Case series in which individuals are followed up over time belong to a different category of research method: the cohort study. For example, a series of diabetic patients were studied to determine the safety of an insulin infusion pump (10). In this study patients were followed for up to 15 months during which time their fasting blood sugar was regularly measured. Most patients found the pump acceptable and many had improved blood sugar control. However, in this case series the element of time over which patients were observed makes this project a cohort study. One of the main concerns with cohort studies is the loss of patients during the follow-up period (other pitfalls are reviewed in Chapter 7). In the infusion pump study 122 patients were initially recruited, but data were only presented for 100 of these. This raises the question of whether poor blood sugar control or dislike of the pump could have contributed to the loss of the other 22 patients. The authors reported that two of these patients had died and others chose not to continue with the study, suggesting that the results obtained may have been biased. Explicit recognition of the type of method being used would simplify the identification of bias, and possibly lead to measures to prevent it.

A Valid Use: Exploration

Having first cautioned about their deficiencies, we can turn to an area in which case series can be used to advantage. They can be used to explore. This could be part of a preliminary enquiry to investigate whether a proposed research study is likely to be successful. Suppose a study wanted to determine why some children are not vaccinated against measles. It would be worth reviewing a small series to clarify whether parents and health care staff of non-vaccinated children could be contacted and would be likely to cooperate by answering questions. This exploration is seeking to answer two questions: Can we do it? Is it worth doing?

Exploration can also involve a more detailed investigation of the beliefs and attitudes of selected persons. Here the intention is to uncover the range of issues, and the different perspectives and motives which affect behaviour. Sometimes this can be an end in itself, and such studies are discussed in Chapter 10 in the section on qualitative methods. In other instances the exploration is part of the preparatory work for a study in which cases are collected in a much more systematic way. For example, in a study of why some women fail to attend for cervical screening, a series of investigative interviews was undertaken (11). These showed the types of costs and benefits which women associated with cervical screening and the barriers that deterred their attendance. This preliminary work was then followed by a larger-scale study which investigated the proportions of women who held the various beliefs and attitudes and assessed their relative importance in determining behaviour (12). In general, exploratory approaches are unhelpful when the interest lies in obtaining estimates of how often certain beliefs are held or how important certain problems are.

COMMENT

Case reports can be useful in showing that unusual events happened, or that expected events did not happen. However, an unusual event may have occurred, but it might be so rare as to have little practical significance. Case reports are also highly susceptible to bias arising from the way the cases were obtained.

Case series are equally susceptible to bias from the way the cases were obtained. Because they are sometimes other methods in disguise (e.g. surveys or cohort studies), they are also subject to the pitfalls and limitations of these methods. Instead of collecting a series it would be better to review the research methods described in Chapters 6 to 10 so that the appropriate design can be selected. Findings based on case reports and case series should be treated with caution bordering on suspicion.

REFERENCES

1. Duchin, JS, Koster, FT, Peters, CJ, et al. Hantavirus pulmonary syndrome: a clinical description of 17 patients with a newly recognized disease. New England Journal of Medicine 1994; 330(14): 949–55.
2. Herbst, AL and Scully, RE. Adenocarcinoma of the vagina in adolescence. A report of 7 cases including 6 clear-cell carcinomas (so-called mesonephromas). Cancer 1970; 25: 745–57.
3. Smith, JC, Cranston, D, O'Brien, T, Guillebaud, J, Hindmarsh, J and Turner,

AG. Fatherhood without apparent spermatozoa after vasectomy. *Lancet* 1994; **344**: 30.

4. Sanchez-Guerra, J, Colditz, GA, Karlson, EW, *et al*. Silicone breast implants and the risk of connective-tissue diseases and symptoms. *New England Journal of Medicine* 1995; **332**: 1666–70.

5. Sackett, DL, Haynes, RB, Guyatt, GH and Tugwell, P. *Clinical Epidemiology: A Basic Science for Clinical Medicine* 2nd edn. Boston, Massachusetts: Little, Brown and Company, 1991: p360.

6. Ruffin, JM, Grizzle, JE, Hightower, NC, McHardy, G, Shull, H and Kirsner, JB. A co-operative double-blind evaluation of gastric "freezing" in the treatment of duodenal ulcer. *New England Journal of Medicine* 1969; **281**(1): 16–19.

7. Should we case-control? [editorial]. *Lancet* 1990; **335**: 1127–8.

8. Moses, LE. The series of consecutive cases as a device for assessing outcomes of intervention. *New England Journal of Medicine* 1984; **311**(11): 705–10.

9. Neale, G. Clinical analysis of 100 medicolegal cases. *British Medical Journal* 1993; **307**: 1483–7.

10. Mecklenburg, RS, Benson, JW Jr, Becker, NM, *et al*. Clinical use of the insulin infusion pump in 100 patients with Type I diabetes. *New England Journal of Medicine* 1982; **307**(9): 513–18.

11. Orbell, S. Personal comunication.

12. Orbell, S, Crombie, I, Robertson, A, Johnston, G and Kenicer, M. Assessing the effectiveness of a screening campaign: who is missed by eighty percent cervical screening coverage? *Journal of the Royal Society of Medicine* 1995; **88**: 389–94.

Chapter 6

SURVEYS

All health services research involves gathering information, and the survey is one systematic method of doing this. Surveys are very widely used in health services research. They come in a variety of guises, because they can tackle many different types of research question. This chapter reviews the range of uses of surveys and describes how they may be designed to provide useful information cheaply, while avoiding the major pitfalls.

RANGE OF USES

A common use of surveys is to determine the amount of disease and disability that exists either in the community as a whole, or among particular groups within it. Surveys have been used to determine the prevalence of asthma in the population (1), the extent of visual disability in the elderly (2), and the levels of blood pressure among Bengali immigrants in East London (3). Often the surveys look beyond describing the amount of disease to ask why particular events have happened. The types of questions being asked include: Why do some women have abortions? (4); Why do patients fail to keep out-patient appointments? (5) Why are some pregnant women susceptible to rubella infection? (6) Why is chest disease so common in South Wales? (7).

Surveys can also investigate problems with the provision and use of equipment, such as beds, catheters, bandages, or scalpels. For example, one study investigated the availability and state of readiness of essential cardiopulmonary resuscitation equipment (8). It found that many of the emergency trolleys contained unnecessary items and only 9% complied with stated policy.

Another type of question which surveys ask is whether all groups within society have equal and satisfactory access to health care services. Some studies have investigated the uptake of medical care by different

Table 6.1 Range of uses of surveys

Target group	Examples of topics of interest
Patients	Need for services Satisfaction with care given Side effects of care Compliance with therapy Quality of life Health behaviour and beliefs
Health professionals	Knowledge and experience Activities undertaken Attitudes to the provision of care Sources of stress and dissatisfaction Educational needs
Relatives and carers	Understanding of illness and its treatment Satisfaction with information given Knowledge of available support services Attitudes to and stresses of caring
General public or selected subgroups	Morbidity/quality of life Unmet need for services Access to services Use of preventive services Health behaviour and beliefs
Health care facilities	Availability of equipment Staffing levels Training and experience of staff Extent of provision of services Nature of service organisation

social class groups (9), and by single mothers (10). Considerable attention has also been given to whether patients' gender or age influenced the provision of care (11–13).

The delivery of health care is strongly dependent on the attitudes and beliefs of health care providers and patients. Thus surveys have investigated doctors' attitudes to requests for euthanasia (14); the views of asthmatic patients on the medication they take (15); the factors affecting parents' decisions to consult a doctor about their child's respiratory illness (16); and the psychological effects of being offered choice of surgery for breast cancer (17).

These examples show that surveys can be carried out among different groups—from health care professionals to patients and their carers. Surveys can be used to investigate all aspects of service delivery, as well as the attitudes and beliefs of those involved in health care. Table 6.1

reviews these many uses of surveys, arranging them by the target group to be investigated. The wealth of questions which can be answered reflect the power of surveys as a method for health services research.

DESIGN MATTERS

Surveys involve taking samples and collecting data on those included in the sample. Issues of data collection are common to all the methods for health services research, and these are therefore dealt with separately in Chapter 13. This chapter deals solely with the processes and problems of drawing samples. Samples are taken because it is seldom possible to contact everyone in a group. Suppose a survey was being planned to investigate the views of general practitioners about the provision of thrombolytic therapy in the community. It would be very time consuming to solicit the views of all registered GPs, and fortunately it would not be necessary. A sample of GPs would be sufficient to obtain a very good idea of what GPs in general think. Statistical theory shows that a well chosen sample can accurately reflect the views of the whole group. To be able to make general statements with confidence, the sample needs to be drawn with care. The procedures which need to be followed are:

- describe the groups of interest
- obtain a list of possible participants
- decide the sample size
- select the method of sampling

Describe the Groups of Interest

Drawing a sample is the end result of a process which involves three other groups of individuals. These are illustrated in Figure 6.1, and will be discussed using the example of a survey of hospital patients. This study investigated their views on the treatment they had received (18). It was designed to determine the general views of inpatients throughout Britain, but clearly not all of these could be surveyed. Instead patients were recruited from 36 NHS hospitals across the country. Thus we have the distinction between the wider group of interest and the possible study participants (Figure 6.1). Not all the patients at the selected hospitals could be surveyed, and it was decided to collect data on 160 consecutively discharged patients from each hospital (5760 patients overall). This group represents the sample chosen for study. In practice

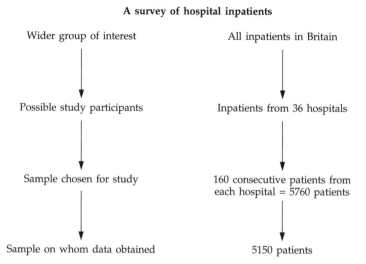

A survey of hospital inpatients

Wider group of interest · All inpatients in Britain

Possible study participants · Inpatients from 36 hospitals

Sample chosen for study · 160 consecutive patients from each hospital = 5760 patients

Sample on whom data obtained · 5150 patients

Figure 6.1   The groups to review when drawing a sample. See Ref. (18)

it was difficult to interview all members of the chosen group. Some of the patients died and others refused to consent or could not be contacted, so that data were actually obtained on 5150 patients.

The importance of the distinctions shown in Figure 6.1 is that they clarify the extent to which generalisations can be made from the sample on whom data are obtained. For example, in the patient survey, care was taken to ensure that the 36 NHS hospitals were representative of (i.e. broadly similar to) all NHS hospitals across the country. Similarly, the intention was to recruit consecutively discharged patients in an attempt to make them representative of all patients seen in those hospitals. The intention was to try to draw a representative sample at each of the steps: i.e. to ensure that the sample on whom data are obtained are likely to be similar to the wider group of interest. If this is achieved, generalisations can be made from the final sample all the way back to all patients seen in NHS hospitals. This process of extrapolation may not be valid if representativeness has not been attained at any of the steps.

In health services research the list of possible participants which is used may not be strictly representative of the broad group of interest. Research is frequently carried out on a local basis, and local lists are used because they are easily obtained. For example, a survey of general practitioners' awareness of vaccine storage conditions was based on clinics in the Manchester area (19). This list was provided by the Central Manchester Health Authority. In theory it would have been possible to sample from lists provided by other health authorities, but this would have substantially increased the workload. The researchers may also have thought that a study conducted by local health care professionals (one of the researchers was a local GP) would encourage a higher response rate. But the key question is whether the finding that only a minority of GPs *were aware of appropriate storage conditions for vaccines* has wider implications. The authors of the report clearly thought so, because they made general recommendations about the provision of adequate equipment and the training of staff in maintaining the cold chain.

The problems of generalisation will always apply to locally based studies. If an atypical group were obtained then the information from the study would relate only to the individuals studied. To be able to extrapolate the results, the researchers must be sure that the group being studied is similar to other groups elsewhere. In the case of the vaccine storage study this would be approached by asking questions of the form: Where do these GPs come from? What are they like? Are they like GPs in other areas? Answering these questions will help clarify the true nature of the group being studied and indicate the extent to which generalisations can be made. If the study group is thought to be unusual, another group could be chosen to make the sample more representative of the wider group.

Obtain a List of Possible Participants

In many instances the group of interest will be too large for everyone to be studied, and a sample will have to be taken from it. This can be most easily achieved when there is an accurate list of the individuals from which the sample can be drawn. This ensures that no one is overlooked, and that all persons can have an equal chance of being included. Somewhat different approaches are taken to obtain lists of health care professionals, patients and members of the general community.

Health Care Professionals

Health care professionals are among the easiest of groups to contact because they are listed in registers of professional bodies, as well as in staff lists of the institutions in which they work. Thus to assess consultant views on the management of myocardial infarction in Scotland, Hutchison and Cobbe (20) used the membership list of the Scottish Society of Physicians because it included most Scottish physicians. The list might not have been complete, but the researchers must have felt that its omissions were unlikely to affect seriously the validity of their conclusions. In other circumstances the omissions could be important and other approaches would be needed to overcome the possible limitations. Thus a survey of pain clinics in Scotland used as a starting point the list of consultant anaesthetist members of the North British Pain Association (21). But because of the rapid development of pain relief clinics it was recognised that there could be important omissions from the list. Therefore, for those hospitals where no consultant anaesthetist was found to be a member of the Association, a questionnaire was sent to one of the anaesthetists listed in the hospital register. The hospitals were identified from the Medical Register.

In some circumstances a list may not be available, or it may be organised such that it is difficult to use. When Philp and colleagues wanted to determine what ward nursing staff thought of the types of care given to the elderly in hospital, they found that the staff could be most easily identified by visiting the long-term care wards and interviewing the staff on duty (22). This ensured that only staff working with the elderly would be contacted. So long as care is taken to sample at different times of day to ensure that staff on shiftwork are covered, this method should work well.

Patients

Selected patient groups can often be identified easily because their contacts with health care may be recorded in a number of different locations. Table 6.2 summarises the variety of sources of patient groups. Computerised registers abound in the health service and they can be a very convenient source of patients. This is well illustrated by a study of coronary catheterisation. The researchers were interested in whether the gender of the patient influenced the chances of having this operation (23). All patients with a diagnosis of ischaemic heart disease were identified from the record of hospital discharges (contained in the Regional Information Database; the Database also recorded the types of operations the patients had had). The study found that women were only half as likely to have coronary catheterisation as men, although the authors stopped short of attributing this to sex discrimination (because they could not exclude the possibility that the effect resulted from differing patterns of disease presentation and progression among women).

Table 6.2 Sources of cases

Setting	Method of identification	Patient characteristics
General practice	Casenote search, repeat prescribing records, register of screening	Mix of severity, many with mild or early stage of disease
Outpatient clinic	Clinic list, outpatient records	Many severe, and often with less common presentations which make diagnosis difficult
Inpatient	Discharge records, laboratory records, cancer registry, pharmacy records, theatre lists	Many severe and acute disease, often with other problems (personal circumstances as well as medical) which have led to hospitalisation
Specialist centre	As inpatient	Predominantly severe cases, many of which have not responded to first-line therapies

In some instances the list of possible study participants is chosen so that the study can be conducted quickly and easily, even although a representative sample may not be obtained. The important point is that the unrepresentativeness does not preclude valid conclusions from being drawn. For example, Gooptu and Mulley (24), wanted to know whether anecdotal reports of elderly people being stuck in baths might indicate that a serious and widespread problem existed. To survey the elderly in the general population would have been a formidable task, involving finding the names and addresses and ages of a sample of people, and contacting them to elicit the information. Instead, the authors surveyed inpatients and those attending the geriatric day hospital during a selected week. They found that most of the 147 patients interviewed had experienced difficulty getting out of the bath. One in seven had become stuck, usually requiring assistance to escape. This study confirmed that there is a serious problem, although because of the patient group studied the exact magnitude of it in the general population cannot be determined. The elderly seen in hospital may well experience more problems of mobility than the general population. This example illustrates the use of a survey to document the existence of a problem (as opposed to estimating its magnitude). The weakness in the method of sampling is recognised, and the conclusions are limited accordingly. Unrepresentative samples can be used, but only if the findings are interpreted with due circumspection.

Individuals in the Community

There are a number of strategies which can be used to contact individuals in the community. These include:

- general practitioner registers
- electoral register
- telephone survey
- *ad hoc* methods

General practitioner lists form one of the most useful population registers for community surveys. They have been used to investigate a wide range of topics including the prevalence of asthma and hay fever (1), the blood pressure of Bengali migrants in East London (3), and levels of physical activity among the old living at home (25). The attraction of these lists is that in addition to name and address they contain details of age and sex, so that particular groups of the community can be targeted. The lists can either be accessed through individual general practices, or centrally through Family Practitioner Committees. Because they are so convenient these lists are widely used. This may lead to increasing reluctance among general practitioners to give approval to research studies, because of the inconvenience which they experience. One limitation to these lists is that, because of population mobility, they may not be fully accurate. This problem is most acute in inner cities which have greater population movement (26).

The electoral register forms another potentially useful population list which has been widely used in survey research (27). It is a published document which is held by public libraries, although permission will usually be required to access it. However, the list does not contain information on age or sex and is limited to those aged over 18 years who are entitled and have registered to vote. Thus it will exclude some of those who tried to avoid paying the poll tax (the ill-fated community charge), as well as those who choose not to be registered to vote for other reasons.

The telephone survey is a technique which was developed in the United States where almost every household has a telephone. It has been used in Britain, for example to estimate the prevalence of chronic pain (28). However, there will be certain groups in society who may not have telephones, and their omission could be a problem for certain types of study.

Some target populations can be very difficult to contact, and ingenuity will be needed to create successful strategies. One of the most difficult groups to contact are injecting drug users, who prefer concealment to prosecution. A study of the prevalence of HIV infection among drug users in New Zealand used the busiest needle exchange outlets in six centres throughout the country as a source of volunteers (29). All persons requesting needles were asked to complete an anonymous questionnaire and provide a saliva sample by chewing on cotton wool. Cooperation was obtained from 73% of drug users, and a low prevalence of HIV infection was found.

A study of the health care experience and the health behaviour of Chinese people in Britain was also faced with the lack of a list: this time of Chinese people. However, it was able to take advantage of the observation that 90% of the Chinese in Britain are employed in the catering industry (30). The study was conducted by surveying the employees of randomly selected Chinese takeaways listed in the *Yellow Pages*. Thus an imaginative approach can lead to the identification of what might initially appear to be inaccessible target populations. The key questions however remain: How representative is the group selected for study? How could the method of sampling influence the study findings? These need to be answered before conclusions are drawn.

Select the Method of Sampling

Having identified the target population, the next question is how to select the sample. The main requirement is that the sample should be drawn so that it is likely to be representative of the target population. There are a number of ways of drawing a sample.

Convenience Sampling

Convenience sampling consists of selecting those patients (or casenotes, or whatever) that happen to be easy to get hold of. While this book frequently argues that the easiest method to achieve a task should be selected, sometimes there can be too much of a good thing. Convenience samples are inevitably biased. The factors which make some subjects easy to contact also ensure that these individuals are different from the target population as a whole. For example, it may be convenient to interview patients when the clinic is not busy, restricting the sample to the types of patients who attend at less busy times. Or some casenotes may be sampled because they are readily available, omitting those which are less readily available (e.g. because the patients have died or been admitted to another ward). Convenience sampling may be used for pilot studies (see Chapter 15), or for exploratory work on the types of responses to particular questions. It is of little value for making generalisations about a wider population.

Simple Random Sampling

The simplest valid method of sampling is to draw what is called a simple random sample. Each possible study participant should have an equal chance of being selected for the sample. In essence, this involves allocating each member of the population a unique number, and then drawing numbers randomly from a hat. In practice, hats are not used. Consider drawing a sample of 20 individuals from a population of 1000. All that is needed is 20 numbers in the range 1 to 1000 selected randomly from all possible numbers in this range. This can be achieved using a table of random numbers, which are provided in many statistics textbooks. This process would be a little tedious for larger samples, and most statisticians would generate the required list of random numbers by computer.

Systematic Sampling

In practice, when the target population is large, simple random sampling can be a cumbersome method of obtaining a sample. It can be easier to use systematic sampling. Say a sample of 200 was required from a population of 1000, then it could be obtained by selecting every fifth patient on the list. The only requirement is that the first patient be randomly selected from among the first five. Similarly, if a sample of 100 were required from a population of 5000 then every 50th patient (i.e. 5000 divided by 100) would be selected, starting somewhere between the first and fiftieth patient. Systematic sampling avoids the tedious business of allocating a unique number to each member of the population. It is particularly useful when patient details have been listed on paper or stored on index cards.

Systematic sampling can be used when the researcher has only a rough idea of the size of the target population. Suppose a large filing cabinet were thought to contain about 1500 sets of casenotes, and a sample of 200 was required. To err on the safe side it is best to take what might be a slight underestimate of the target population, say 1400 sets of notes. Thus every seventh set of notes (1400 divided by 200) would be taken, starting at a random point between one and seven. If in the event there were as many as 1600 sets of notes, the resulting sample size would only be a little larger than intended (229 rather than 200). Small deviations in sample size from that originally proposed have no practical effect (unless this results in unusual individuals being selectively lost or selectively included in the sample).

In some circumstances systematic sampling can produce an atypical sample. This occurs when the individuals on the list are arranged in some kind of order. Consider what might happen if a general practitioner's list was used in a survey of familial aggregation of asthma. The list might well be arranged by patient surname, so that all members of a family could be grouped together. Then a systematic sample which selected every tenth person would select a maximum of one representative from each family (except those which contained more than nine persons). In this instance systematic sampling would defeat the aims of the study. Careful review of the consequences of the sampling method should clarify when difficulties are likely to be encountered. In practice, problems are seldom encountered with systematic sampling.

Other Sampling Methods

There are other, more sophisticated, methods of sampling which are particularly suited to populations which fall naturally into a number of groups. For example, if a study was to investigate the opinions of hospital doctors, it might seem sensible to divide them into groups by their level of experience: such as consultants, senior registrars, registrars and so on. Then a sample could be drawn separately from each group. This technique is called stratified sampling: the members of the population are divided into groups (or strata) by some characteristic. (In the example the characteristic was staff seniority, but if studying patients it could be age, duration of disease or severity of disease.) When the whole population has been divided into groups, a sample is drawn from each one. This approach increases the chances of drawing a representative sample. It can also mean that precise estimates can be obtained with smaller sample sizes than would be required for simple random sampling.

Sometimes the population being studied falls into so many groups that it would be inconvenient to sample from every one. For example, general practitioner lists can be a convenient means of sampling individuals from the community. This approach was used to assess blood pressure levels in districts throughout Scotland (31). However, it would have been inconvenient to sample from every GP list in each district. The workload was reduced by first selecting a random sample of GPs, and then drawing a sample from each of their lists. This technique is called cluster sampling. The population is divided into a set of groups or clusters, and a sample of these groups is chosen for more detailed study.

Often within the groups chosen a further sample is taken to obtain the subjects for study.

Stratified sampling and cluster sampling can offer theoretical and practical advantages. But these techniques require special methods for calculating the sample size and for carrying out the analysis. The interested reader could learn more about these methods by referring to the texts listed at the end of this chapter, but would be better advised to discuss these issues with a statistician.

Decide the Sample Size

One problem with surveys is that the samples obtained are subject to the play of chance. Consider a study of doctors' attitudes to euthanasia which found that '46% of doctors would consider taking active steps to bring about the death of a patient if it were legal to do so' (14). It is possible that by chance alone the sample included more (or fewer) in favour of euthanasia than is true for doctors as a whole. The concern then is by how much the play of chance could influence the findings. Fortunately, it is relatively easy to calculate an interval about the sample estimate (46%) which is likely to contain the proportion which would have been obtained had all doctors been asked about euthanasia. In this example with a sample size of 307, it is likely that the true value lies somewhere between 40 and 52%. This interval is the 95% confidence interval, the range within which we are 95% sure that the true value lies. (Confidence intervals are discussed again in Chapter 15.) The interval is calculated using the formula below, where p is the percentage in favour of euthanasia, $100-p$ is the percentage who do not favour it, and n is the size of the sample (32):

$$p \pm 1.96 \times \sqrt{\frac{p \times (100 - p)}{n}}$$

Substituting in the values it becomes:

$$46 \pm 1.96 \times \sqrt{\frac{46 \times (100 - 46)}{307}}$$

$$46 \pm 1.96 \times \sqrt{8.09}$$

$$46 \pm 5.6$$

40 to 52

The multiplier 1.96 is used to give a 95% confidence interval. Other multipliers can be used if we want to be even more certain of including the true value. For example, we would use 2.57 to give a 99% confidence

Table 6.3 Sample size required for estimated proportion to fall in desired range

True value	Desired range	Required sample size
5%	±1%	1 900
5%	±3%	212
20%	±1%	6 400
20%	±3%	712
20%	±5%	256
50%	±1%	10 000
50%	±3%	1 112
50%	±5%	400
50%	±10%	100

interval, in which we would be 99% certain that the true value lay. (These multipliers derive from statistical theory which is beyond the scope of this book.) Note that increasing the certainty of including the true value produces a much wider range (from 37% to 55%). It is because of this that the 95% confidence interval is used as a compromise between being fairly certain of including the true value without having a very wide interval.

The confidence interval approach can be used to decide the size of a survey, by indicating how precise the sample estimate should be. Consider a survey to determine what proportion of stroke patients in the community need some form of home help. If the true proportion was, say, 30%, then a survey of 100 people would most likely give an answer in the range 21% to 39%. This range would seem too large to be useful: it would, for example, be of little use for deciding the amount of extra service provision which would be needed. It might be felt that, whatever the true value, the sample estimate should be within ±5%. In this case the sample would need to contain 336 individuals.

The required sample size for several sets of circumstances is shown in Table 6.3. This table shows the sample size required so that the estimate of the true proportion falls within a specified range. Suppose in reality the true prevalence of undiagnosed asthmatics in the general population were 5%. If the sample estimate was to fall, say, within ±3% of this, then a sample of 212 people would be required. Two rules of thumb emerge from this table: unless a large range of uncertainty is acceptable, samples of less than 200 will be unsuitable; and even with large samples, the estimate of the proportion should not be thought of as exact, as the true proportion could lie a little way on either side. This table is only presented to illustrate the consequences of different sample sizes. Before conducting a survey, an exact sample size should be calculated, either by contacting a statistician or referring to a textbook. A book by Lemeshow and colleagues (33) is devoted to sample size calculations, and one by Bland (34) has a chapter dealing with this issue.

ANALYSIS AND INTERPRETATION

The data produced by surveys are probably the easiest to analyse when compared to the other research methods. The basic approach to data analysis is described in Chapter 15, so this will not be repeated here. Instead, this section will focus on a type of analysis most often carried out in surveys: the calculation of proportions and rates.

Calculating Proportions

Calculating proportions is often a straightforward matter. In a survey of hospital patients (18) the number who experienced pain (3163) was divided by the number of persons who took part in the survey (5150) to obtain 61%. However, in dealing with the question of the number of patients who had to ask for drugs for their pain (1085), the relevant denominator is no longer the total number in the survey. Instead, it is the number who had pain (3136), so the proportion is 1085/3136=42%. Those who did not have pain are excluded from the denominator, because they were never likely to ask for pain medication. This is one instance of the rule for proportions: that all those in the denominator must have had the opportunity to appear in the numerator.

In some instances an inappropriate denominator could be used inadvertently. For example, a review of suicide by ingestion of anti-depressants found that two drugs, amitriptyline and dothiepin, were responsible for 81.6% of deaths (35). However it cannot be concluded these are the most dangerous antidepressant drugs. The calculation using the total number of deaths as the denominator takes no account of the number of people taking each antidepressant. A more appropriate denominator would be the number of prescriptions issued for each drug. When this is used, amitriptyline and dothiepin are found to have moderate fatality rates (deaths per million prescriptions) compared to other tricyclic antidepressants. In general, when calculating a rate it is important to clarify which is the set of subjects at risk of appearing in the numerator, so that the appropriate denominator can be used.

Prevalence and Incidence Rates

Surveys are often used to estimate how common a disease or condition is in a selected group of the community. Thus a survey was carried out to determine the frequency of visual disability in the elderly: it found that among those aged over 65 years, 14.9% reported difficulty in seeing which was not corrected by glasses or contact lenses (2). The interest in this type of survey lies in estimating the number of people with the problem, irrespective of when it first developed. This is the prevalence of the condition. The findings can indicate whether health care needs are being met, and suggest changes that might be required in the organisation and delivery of care.

Surveys provide an estimate of disease prevalence, the number of existing cases of a disease or disability (divided by the population size to provide a rate). The prevalence reflects a balance between the number of cases disappearing from the community (through cure or death) and the number of new cases which occur. Because of this balance, prevalence is less useful in deciding whether a disease is becoming more or less common, whether its frequency is increasing or decreasing. Changes in prevalence could reflect changes in death rates or the development of a new treatment, as well as changes in the number of new cases which occur. Thus to measure changes in disease frequency another measure, the incidence rate, is used. This is the number of new cases which occur over a defined period (often one year), divided by the population size. The incidence rate is much more sensitive to the occurrence of epidemics, but it cannot easily be estimated from a survey. Incidence rates are best calculated from a cohort study (see Chapter 7).

Adjusting Rates for Age and Sex

Rates are often heavily influenced by the age and sex composition of the group being studied. This is most clearly seen in comparisons of death rates in different communities. Alderson (36) gives a good example by comparing the frequency of death between men in the armed forces and farmers. At first sight the annual death rate in the farmers (5.9 per 1000 men) is substantially higher than in the armed forces (2.8 per 1000 men). However, men in the armed forces tend to leave the service at a young age, and only a small proportion continue in employment over the age of 45 years. In contrast, many farmers continue working in their 50s and 60s. As death rates rise rapidly with age we would expect relatively more deaths among the farmers because of the larger proportion of older men. When allowance is made for the difference in age distribution, using a technique known as standardisation, the death rate among farmers is found to be about 20% lower than the national average, whereas that among the armed forces is about 50% higher than the average. The positions on mortality have been reversed.

The technique of standardisation is straightforward, although it is computationally tedious. The details of it are outlined in texts on epidemiology, especially those by Lilienfeld and Lilienfeld (37) and Mausner and Kramer (38).

Age and sex are not the only factors which can influence survey results. For example, a survey of the prevalence of schizophrenia among homeless people found it was necessary to adjust for type of residence and duration of unemployment as well as age (39). In other circumstances it may be necessary to adjust for social factors: for example, there is evidence that social class influences uptake of medical care (9). Adjustment for these factors can be made in the same way as for age and sex.

POTENTIAL PITFALLS

The design of surveys involves sampling and collecting data, so it should come as little surprise that these are the two areas where the pitfalls lie.

Collecting too much Data

Deciding which data items to collect in a survey can be difficult: 'Most surveys suffer from trying to get too much information on too many problems in a single study. This must be avoided at all costs' (40). The way to avoid this problem is to refine the research question and identify the essential data items.

The process of refining the research question involves converting the germ of an idea into a focused research question which indicates what the study intends to find out and how it intends to do so (see Chapter 3). From the refined question a list can be prepared of the areas on which data could be collected. This is compiled by asking: What do I need to measure to answer the research question? As issues of measurement are common to all methods of health services research, they are discussed in more detail in Chapter 13.

Biases in Sampling

All methods in health services research are prone to several sources of bias. The consequence is that the results obtained are systematically different to what is true in reality. The various types of bias and strategies to minimise their effect are reviewed in Chapter 15. However, surveys are particularly vulnerable to problems associated with the way samples are drawn, and these will be covered here. If samples are not drawn with care, they may not be representative of the wider group of interest. The main ways that this can happen are:

- non-coverage
- non-response

Non-coverage

A problem can arise if some members of the target population are never included in the list from which the sample is drawn. This is termed non-coverage. For example, homeless people will often not be included in population registers and thus might not be covered in community surveys of health needs. This becomes important when there is sub-stantial non-coverage and when those not covered differ to those who are covered. In the community survey example, the importance of the homeless is that they are likely to have quite different health needs to those with accommodation. Thus a misleading picture of the overall health needs of the community would be given if there were more than a few percent of homeless in the population. Non-coverage can also occur when surveying objects such as emergency trolleys or fire extinguishers. It is likely that there are good reasons why some pieces of equipment are not on the list. For example, they may be in obscure, out-of-the-way places, and not have been looked at for a considerable time. Whatever the reasons, those not on the list may well differ from the others. The potential for non-coverage bias can be reduced by ensuring that the list from which the sample will be drawn is as up to date and complete as possible.

There is another form of non-coverage which is less evident but which often affects patient surveys. The characteristics of patients depend heavily on the source from which they are obtained (see Table 6.2). In general, the proportion of patients with severe disease will increase from general practice through to specialist referral centres. Patients with other medical conditions or problems (especially other disabilities which need some degree of support) are more likely to be hospitalised. Patients sampled in one setting (e.g. on a ward) are likely to differ systematically from those in other settings (e.g. being cared for at home). In consequence, the conclusions from the survey will be restricted to the types of patients studied.

Non-response

Most surveys find that they are unable to obtain information on a number of those chosen for study. The reasons for this non-response include absence from home at the time of the study as well as refusal to take part. Again, the potential for bias depends on both the number and the nature of non-responders. It is usually worth making some effort to minimise this source of bias. Many studies make up to three attempts to contact members of the sample to reduce the number of non-responders. Surveys of patient groups often have high response rates, perhaps because patients have a feeling of gratitude or even obligation to health care professionals. Surveys of the general population tend to have lower response rates and more attention needs to be given to ways of improving response. People will be more likely to respond when they feel the study is relevant and important to them. Personalised letters can help if they outline the way the study will improve health care and emphasise the importance of the individual's contribution.

There is a view that community surveys can be meaningfully interpreted when the proportion of responders is at least 70%. Although there is no real basis for this, the converse may well be true; that if the response rate falls short of 70% then the study findings may be in doubt. Where possible information should be sought on the non-responders to determine the extent to which they are likely to differ from responders.

In some circumstances a low response rate is unavoidable because the target population is so difficult to contact. This happened in the survey of schizophrenia mentioned above, where it proved difficult to interview many of the homeless people. One way to deal with this is to make a special effort to gain other information about the non-responders. Thus the authors of the schizophrenia study obtained information on the non-responders from a computerised psychiatric register. This showed little evidence of systematic differences between responders and non-responders, so that the findings from the study were not brought into doubt by a low response rate.

COMMENT AND FURTHER READING

Surveys are one of the commonest methods used in health services research. Many types of survey can be readily undertaken and can require only the most modest of resources. Even large numbers of persons can be contacted in a short period for a comparatively small cost if postal questionnaires are used. When designed and conducted with care, surveys can produce valid findings which are easily interpreted. Thus the survey can be a good method to choose—if there is a research question which is interesting and worthwhile, and suited to investigation by survey.

Survey sampling can be a sophisticated business and there are a number of textbooks devoted to it. Two classical texts by Moser and Kalton (27) and Kish (41) are general works on survey sampling. More recent books by Cartwright (42) and Abramson (43) deal solely with health surveys. A publication from the King's Fund gives a detailed and very readable description of all the stages in the design and conduct of a survey of the last year of life of a sample of adults (44). Two introductory statistics textbooks provide chapters on the various methods of sampling (45, 46). Those wishing to explore the more theoretical aspects of sampling could try the more advanced books by Barnett (47) and Cochran (48).

REFERENCES

1. Fleming, DM and Crombie, DL. Prevalence of asthma and hay fever in England and Wales. *British Medical Journal* 1987; **294**: 279–83.
2. Harries, U, Landes, R and Popay, J. Visual disability among older people: a case study in assessing needs and examining services. *Journal of Public Health Medicine* 1994; **16**(2): 211–18.
3. Silman, AJ, Evans, SJW and Loysen, E. Blood pressure and migration: a study of Bengali immigrants in East London. *Journal of Epidemiology and Community Health* 1987; **41**: 152–5.
4. Houghton, A. Women who have abortions—are they different? *Journal of Public Health Medicine* 1994; **16**(3): 296–304.
5. Andrews, R, Morgan, JD, Addy, DP and McNeish, AS. Understanding non-attendance in outpatient paediatric clinics. *Archives of Diseases in Childhood* 1990; **65**: 192–5.
6. Lawman, S, Morton, K and Best, JM. Reasons for rubella susceptibility among pregnant women in West Lambeth. *Journal of the Royal Society of Medicine* 1994; **87**: 263–4.
7. Burr, ML and Holliday, RM. Why is chest disease so common in South Wales? Smoking, social class, and lung function: a survey of elderly men in two areas. *Journal of Epidemiology and Community Health* 1987; **41**: 140–4.
8. Campbell, J. Cardio pulmonary resuscitation—audit of emergency trolleys. In: Bain, J, Crombie, IK and Davies, HTO, eds. *Clinical Audit Occasional Papers: Audit Symposium 1993*. Edinburgh: HMSO, 1993.
9. Balarajan, R, Yuen, P and Machin, D. Socioeconomic differentials in the uptake of medical care in Great Britain. *Journal of Epidemiology and Community Health* 1987; **41**: 196–9.

10. Beatson-Hird, P, Yuen, P and Balarajan, R. Single mothers: their health and health service use. *Journal of Epidemiology and Community Health* 1989; **43**: 385–90.
11. Petticrew, M, McKee, M and Jones, J. Coronary artery surgery: are women discriminated against? *British Medical Journal* 1993; **306**: 1164–6.
12. Clarke, KW, Gray, D, Keating, NA and Hampton, JR. Do women with acute myocardial infarction receive the same treatment as men? *British Medical Journal* 1994; **309**: 563–6.
13. Hannaford, PC, Kay, CR and Ferry, S. Ageism as explanation for sexism in provision of thrombolysis. *British Medical Journal* 1994; **309**: 573.
14. Ward, BJ and Tate, PA. Attitudes among NHS doctors to requests for euthanasia. *British Medical Journal* 1994; **308**: 1332–4.
15. Osman, LM, Russell, IT, Friend, JAR, Legge, JS and Douglas, JG. Predicting patient attitudes to asthma medication. *Thorax* 1993; **48**(8): 827–30.
16. Wyke, S, Hewison, J and Russell, IT. Respiratory illness in children: what makes parents decide to consult? *British Journal of General Practice* 1990; **40**: 226–9.
17. Fallowfield, LJ, Hall, A, Maguire, P, Baum, M and A'Hern, RP. Psychological effects of being offered choice of surgery for breast cancer. *British Medical Journal* 1994; **309**: 448.
18. Bruster, S, Jarman, B, Bosanquet, N, Weston, D, Erens, R and Delbanco, TL. National survey of hospital patients. *British Medical Journal* 1994; **309**: 1542–6.
19. Thakker, Y and Woods, S. Storage of vaccines in the community: weak link in the cold chain? *British Medical Journal* 1992; **304**: 756–8.
20. Hutchison, SJ and Cobbe, SM. Management of myocardial infarction in Scotland: have clinical trials changed practice? *British Medical Journal* 1987; **294**: 1261.
21. Bisset, WIK. Pain relief clinics under anaesthetic management in Scotland. *Annals of the Royal College of Surgeons England* 1988; **70**: 392–4.
22. Philp, I, Mawhinney, S and Mutch, WJ. Setting standards for long term care of the elderly in hospital. *British Medical Journal* 1991; **302**: 1056.
23. Kee, F, Gaffney, B, Currie, S and O'Reilly, D. Access to coronary catheterisation: fair shares for all? *British Medical Journal* 1993; **307**: 1305–7.
24. Gooptu, C, Mulley, GP. Survey of elderly people who get stuck in the bath. *British Medical Journal* 1994; **308**: 762.
25. Dallosso, HM, Morgan, K, Bassey, EJ, Ebrahim, SBJ, Fentem, PH and Arie, THD. Levels of customary physical activity among the old and the very old living at home. *Journal of Epidemiology and Community Health* 1988; **42**: 121–7.
26. Bowling, A, Hart, D and Silman, A. Accuracy of electoral registers and family practitioner committee lists for population studies of the very elderly. *Journal of Epidemiology and Community Health* 1989; **43**: 391–4.
27. Moser, CA and Kalton, G. *Survey Methods in Social Investigation* 2nd edn. London: Heinemann Educational Books, 1971.
28. Bowsher, D, Rigge, M, and Sopp, L. Prevalence of chronic pain in the British population: a telephone survey of 1037 households. *The Pain Clinic* 1991; **4**(4): 223–30.
29. Dickson, NP, Austin, FJ, Paul, C, Sharples, KJ and Skegg, DCG. HIV surveillance by testing saliva from injecting drug users: a national study in New Zealand. *Journal of Epidemiology and Community Health* 1994; **48**: 55–7.
30. Watt, IS, Howel, D and Lo, L. The health care experience and health

behaviour of the Chinese: a survey based in Hull. *Journal of Public Health Medicine* 1993; **15**(2): 129–36.

31. Crombie, IK, Smith, WCS, Tavendale, R and Tunstall-Pedoe, H. Geographical clustering of risk factors and lifestyle for coronary heart disease in the Scottish Heart Health Study. *British Heart Journal* 1990; **64**: 199–203.

32. Gardner, MJ and Altman, DJ. *Statistics with Confidence*. London: British Medical Journal, 1990.

33. Lemeshow, S, Hosmer, DW Jr, Klar, J and Lwanga, SK. *Adequacy of Sample Size in Health Studies*. Chichester: John Wiley & Sons, 1990.

34. Bland, N. *An Introduction to Medical Statistics* 2nd edn. Oxford: Oxford University Press, 1995.

35. Henry, JA, Alexander, CA and Sener, EK. Relative mortality from overdose of antidepressants. *British Medical Journal* 1995; **310**: 221–4.

36. Alderson, M. *An Introduction to Epidemiology* 2nd edn. London: Macmillan Press, 1983.

37. Lilienfeld, AM and Lilienfeld, DE. *Foundations of Epidemiology* 2nd edn. New York: Oxford University Press, 1980.

38. Mausner, JS, Kramer, S. *Mausner & Bahn. Epidemiology: An Introductory Text* 2nd edn. Philadelphia: W B Saunders Company, 1985.

39. Geddes, J, Newton, R, Young, G, Bailey, S, Freeman, C and Priest, R. Comparison of prevalence of schizophrenia among residents of hostels for homeless people in 1966 and 1992. *British Medical Journal* 1994; **308**: 816–19.

40. World Health Organization. *Planning and Organising a Health Survey*. Geneva: World Health Organization, 1981: p14.

41. Kish, L. *Survey Sampling*. New York: John Wiley & Sons, 1965.

42. Cartwright, A. *Health Surveys in Practice and in Potential: A Critical Review of their Scope and Methods*. London: King Edward's Hospital Fund for London, 1983.

43. Abramson, JH. *Survey Methods in Community Medicine: Epidemiological Studies, Programme Evaluation, Clinical Trials* 4th edn. Edinburgh: Churchill Livingstone, 1990.

44. Cartwright, A and Seale, C. *The Natural History of a Survey: An Account of the Methodological Issues Encountered in a Study of Life Before Death*. London: King Edward's Hospital Fund for London, 1990.

45. Daly, J, McDonald, I and Willis, E, eds. *Researching Health Care. Designs, Dilemmas, Disciplines*. London: Tavistock/Routledge, 1992.

46. Weiss, NA and Hassett, MJ. *Introductory Statistics* 2nd edn. Reading, Massachusetts: Addison-Wesley, 1987.

47. Barnett, V. *Elements of Sampling Theory*. London: Hodder and Stoughton, 1986.

48. Cochran, WG. *Sampling Techniques* 3rd edn. New York: John Wiley & Sons, 1977.

Chapter 7

COHORT STUDIES

The cohort study is the research method concerned with observing events over time, to provide valid answers to questions of the form: How well did these patients fare? What was their subsequent use of health care resources? It is a research method which has been comparatively little used in health services research, but future years are likely to see a considerable increase in the frequency of its use. This reflects the change in the focus of medicine from a predominant concern with the immediate outcome of therapy, to one of greater attention to the longer-term well-being of patients.

The term cohort derives from a Latin word for a body of soldiers. As a cohort of soldiers can be envisioned marching along a straight Roman road, so a cohort of patients can be imagined passing through time. This chapter describes the range of uses of cohort studies, and reviews key elements of their design and analysis.

RANGE OF USES

Cohort studies can be used in a variety of ways in health services research, including to:

• determine whether patients need long term follow-up
• detect long-term adverse effects of medical interventions
• investigate continued health care usage
• evaluate patient well-being in the longer term
• clarify the natural history of a disease

In many settings patients are seen over a limited period, possibly a few weeks or months. Although they may be successfully managed in the short term, the longer-term needs for health care may remain unknown. Concern about the longer-term well-being of patients may lead to their being given regular follow-up appointments. However, the key question is whether this extended follow-up can be justified. Patients with photosensitivity dermatitis and actinic reticuloid syndrome illustrate the problem. There was suspicion that many of these patients would develop a malignant cutaneous lymphoma (1). If this were true, the patients would need regular lifelong follow-up appointments so that the cancers could be detected at an early stage. However, if the opposing view were correct, that the photodermatitis lesions were sometimes misdiagnosed as lymphomas, the lifetime follow-up would be a substantial waste of resources. The issue was resolved by identifying a set of photodermatitis patients and tracking them for many years to determine how many developed a lymphoma. Of 231 patients followed up, six had a diagnosis of lymphoma, and detailed inspection of the clinical notes showed that all but one of these had the photodermatitis misdiagnosed as lymphoma. This study was able to confirm that that there was no substantial increase in lymphoma risk, and indeed if there were an increased risk it must be very small. This study illustrates the basic features of cohort studies: identify a group of patients and follow them over time to see what happens.

There is a general concern in medicine that procedures which appear valuable may have unforeseen long-term adverse effects. The thalidomide disaster is one which drew attention to the potential long-term hazards of drugs, and there have now been many studies investigating these hazards. Adverse effects are not limited to drugs and other procedures in medicine have been studied. For example, the risk of developing testicular cancer following vasectomy was investigated by studying 74 000 Danish men who had had the operation (there was no increased risk of developing the cancer) (2).

Another way in which cohort studies can be used is in monitoring the long-term use of health care facilities. For example, one researcher investigated changes in drug use among the elderly over a 10-year period (3). The study confirmed the suspected increase in the consumption of drugs, particularly vitamins and analgesics.

For many chronic diseases the long-term prognosis is only poorly understood. Yet a question which patients with these diseases often ask is: How well will I be in five or ten years' time? To be able to counsel patients or their carers, detailed information is needed on the likely outcomes. One striking example of this is cerebral palsy in children, where until recently there was 'little information on life expectancy' (4). A recent cohort study which followed 1251 children with idiopathic cerebral palsy found that survival was better than was previously thought: over 85% lived for at least 20 years from diagnosis (4).

DESIGN MATTERS

The defining characteristic of the cohort study is that it involves the follow-up of patients over time. It is really a form of survey to which the element of time has been added. As such, it is subject to the same design constraints and pitfalls as surveys. But to obtain valid results there are many other features of study design which should be considered. For most applications in health services research, the design considerations which apply are:

- specify the study group
- set the follow-up period
- measure the outcome
- speed up the follow-up
- determine the sample size

Specify the Study Group

The design of cohort studies begins with a clear specification of the patient group to be investigated. This process should answer the question: Who exactly are we going to study? This in turn will depend on clarifying: What do we want to find out? The general nature of the group of patients to be studied will often be obvious from the research question. But the study group needs to be specified in detail giving: the criteria for diagnosis; the setting from which patients are to be obtained; and the time period over which patients are to be recruited. For example, a study of mortality among epileptics focused on newly diagnosed cases, where epilepsy was defined by the occurrence of one or more seizures (5). Neonatal seizures and patients previously diagnosed as epileptic were excluded. The patients were obtained from 275 participating general practices throughout the UK, and were recruited over the period 1984–7. This extended recruitment period reflects the slow rate at which new cases of epilepsy present in general practice.

When specifying the study group, attention needs to be given to how the members of the group will be identified. One method of identifying patients is by trawling through sets of casenotes. This would identify those who have the disease or have received the treatment which is the focus of study. But this can be a tedious business. Fortunately there are several other ways of identifying patients, and these are listed in Table 6.2 in Chapter 6. As usual the source is selected to yield sufficient numbers of patients most easily. Sometimes no single source will be sufficient and several will need to be used. Thus a study of the long-term management of children with sickle cell disease used four separate sources because there was no register of affected children (6). These were hospital discharge records, an outpatient register, a ward diagnostic register and the records of the haematology department. The study found several deficiencies in care, for example *'prophylactic treatment with penicillin and folic acid was erratic'*, and recommended a more systematic approach to long-term management.

Set the Follow-up Period

The question: How long should patients be followed-up for? is one that requires careful consideration. For example, if the interest lay in determining the life expectancy of a group of patients, many years of follow-up would be required. This is why the study of life expectancy of children with cerebral palsy mentioned above followed children with the disease for up to 27 years (4). However, in health services research the follow-up period will seldom last this long. Thus a study which investigated the effect of the type of infant feeding (bottle or breast) on subsequent morbidity observed babies for up to two years after birth (7). In some circumstances the follow-up period will only be a few days. For example, a study of morbidity following day-case laparoscopy was interested in events immediately following surgery, and thus observed side effects for two days after the operation (8).

These examples show that the general answer to the question: How long? is long enough to detect the relevant effects. The period may be relatively short, or may extend for several years. In practice, the follow-up period will often be limited by the resources available. Then the study should only be undertaken if the correct answer is obtained to the question: Is it likely that enough events of interest will have occurred during the period of observation?

Measure the Outcome

One of the major difficulties of cohort studies is determining the outcome at the end of follow-up. There are two problems: how to contact the patient after time has elapsed; and how to determine the outcome. Achieving both can be straightforward when the study involves hospital inpatients and the outcome can be assessed before discharge. For example, the occurrence of adverse events such as bed sores could be determined by inspection while the patient is still in hospital. But once patients have been discharged, follow-up is much more difficult. Several strategies are available to obtain the necessary data:

- casenotes
- routinely collected data
- postal questionnaire
- home interview
- NHS central register

For many topics the required outcome data can be obtained from the casenotes so that follow-up can be achieved simply by reviewing the notes. This was the method used to determine the management which the children with sickle cell disease had received. But casenote data can have deficiencies which limit their usefulness: the notes themselves may not always be available, and the data they contain may be incomplete or inaccurate. For the sickle cell study described above, the problem of deficiencies in casenotes was less acute than it could be in other circumstances. It focused on discrete events, such as attendance at outpatient clinics, which are likely to be recorded. Other items, like the information given to patients, may be absent.

There are many sources of routinely collected data which could be used to assess outcome (see Chapter 10). Discharge diagnoses on hospital inpatients are a valuable source of follow-up data. They have been used to investigate whether adverse events follow the administration of tagamet (9), to assess mortality following surgery (10), and to measure readmission rates of discharged patients (11). These sources need to be used with care because of concerns about the accuracy of the data they contain (12–14).

A postal questionnaire to discharged patients is one of the easiest methods of follow-up. This approach was used in a study of post-operative wound infection to determine whether wound infection could develop after discharge (15). The researchers found several cases of previously unsuspected infections among patients who had undergone general and orthopaedic surgery. Postal questionnaires are very susceptible to non-response. It is likely that non-responders will be different in kind to those who respond. One factor which will encourage a high response is emphasising the relevance of the study to the participants. The use of postal questionnaires is also limited by the propensity which some people have to move home. The longer the interval since the last contact with health care, the greater the proportion who will have moved and thus cannot be contacted. Population turnover is much more of a problem in the major cities than in rural areas.

Interviews with patients, often in their own homes, provide a more flexible and sensitive method of data collection than postal questionnaires. This approach has been used for a range of studies, including the use of health care services following stroke (16) and the types of residence of discharged psychotic patients (17). As with postal questionnaires, this type of study can be affected by population movement if a substantial period has occurred since patients were last seen by health professionals. However, it is possible to carry out extended follow-ups if special efforts are made to find patients. Thus the study of discharged psychotic patients carried out a careful tracing exercise using records of contact with psychiatric services, general practitioner records and the police.

One of the most effective methods of following patients through time is the NHS central register. This register was set up at the start of the Second World War as means of registering the population of Britain. When the NHS was established in 1948, GPs were paid according to the number of patients on their lists. The wartime register was a convenient means for organising this payment and for tracking patients when they moved home. There is a financial incentive for GPs to register new patients and for health authorities to remove patients who have moved, emigrated or died. Thus the register is kept up to date.

The register provides a means of identifying which patients have died and the dates and causes of death. One study monitored the survival of patients with Alzheimer's disease to investigate suggestions that these patients had a reduced life expectancy (18). This was confirmed: on average patients lived for only 69% of the time expected. The register can also be used to identify the health area in which a patient lives, so that the appropriate Family Health Service Authority can be approached for permission to contact the patient's doctor. The register was computerised in 1991 so that patients can be traced more quickly and cheaply. The key to the system is a valid patient NHS number, and in 1995 it only cost 65p to trace each patient with this information. Those wishing to use the register can obtain further information and an application form from:

Health Statistics
OPCS
10 Kingsway
London WC2B 6JP

Speed up the Follow-up

Often the interest of a study lies with the long-term outcome, but few researchers can sit about for years until the results become interesting. The alternative is to identify the patients from the past, going back several years if necessary. These patients can then be followed up to the present day. This was the method chosen for a study of the long-term outcome of schizophrenia. The disease is popularly viewed as *'a chronic deteriorating illness making long term demands on services and creating an almost intolerable burden for relatives and carers'* (17). To investigate this, a set of patients first seen between 1978 and 1980 were identified from records and traced and interviewed to determine their current status (an average of 13 years of follow-up). The results challenge the accepted view: most patients were living independently and many had no contact with psychiatric services.

Using cases from many years in the past increases the difficulty of tracing patients. After 13 years many patients will have moved house. The difficulty will be compounded for patients with chronic diseases, many of whom may be forced to move to some form of sheltered accommodation. It is in circumstances like these that the NHS central register becomes an invaluable tool for cohort studies.

Determine the Sample Size

The sample size for a cohort study is often limited by the number of patients available for study. However, rather than just hoping that the available number will be sufficient, it is better to check at the outset that the number is large enough to make the study worthwhile. Formal sample size calculations should be carried out. Methods are presented in papers by Cutler and colleagues (19) and Schlesselman (20) and books by Lemeshow and colleagues (21) and Breslow and Day (22). Before these are read, or a statistician contacted for advice, some rules of thumb may be helpful. When cohort studies investigate common events, for example those that are expected to occur in 10–20% of patients, then a study size of about 100 will often be adequate. The study of schizophrenic patients described above obtained valuable results with 99 patients. However when the outcome of interest is less common, occurring in, say, 2–3% of subjects, then a sample of several hundred would be required. If the outcome of interest (e.g. development of cancer) is rare, then a very large study would be required. For example, it would take several thousand subjects to detect events which only occurred among one individual in 500. Cohort studies need to be large to study rare outcomes, and other methods such as the case-control study (see Chapter 9) should be considered.

ANALYSIS AND INTERPRETATION

The analysis of cohort studies can involve little more than calculating the proportion of patients who exhibit some characteristic at the end of the follow-up period. For example, duodenal ulcer can be caused by *Helicobacter pylori*, and this is treated by the eradication of the infective agent. However, the unresolved question is whether patients remain free from infection over the longer term. A cohort study showed 92% of patients remained *H. pylori* negative after an average follow-up period of 7.1 years (23). Studies which can use this simple form of analysis are those which are concerned with the broad picture, seeking answers of the form: Does this event occur frequently or rarely in the study group?

Comparison Groups

In some circumstances it can be difficult to interpret the findings from cohort studies. Consider a study carried out to determine whether amniocentesis has any long-term adverse effects on children born after this procedure. The offspring of 1300 women who had had amniocentesis were followed for up to 18 years and 128 were found to have some form of disability or handicap (24). How would one interpret this observation? Some cases of disability or handicap would be expected to occur even if the women had not had an amniocentesis. The issue then is how to decide whether more adverse events were occurring than would be expected. This was resolved by determining the frequency of disability or handicap among a control group of children, matched by sex, date and place of birth and by age of the mother. This showed that the frequency of adverse events was very similar in the two groups (9.9% of the amniocentesis mothers and 8.3% of the controls).

In studies which use a comparison group, great care must be taken that the controls really are comparable with the study group. The amniocentesis study described above carefully matched the controls to the study group on several factors. When comparison groups are used, the overriding concern is whether subtle differences between the study group and the controls could influence the findings. In some circumstances it is possible to adjust for differences between the groups in the analysis. For example, Howie and colleagues (7) were interested in the effect of breast feeding on gastrointestinal infection. They wanted to follow up the babies of mothers who chose to breast feed and compare the frequency of infection against babies who were bottle fed. But they were concerned that the two groups might differ in factors like parental social class, parental smoking and maternal age. These factors were found to influence the risk of infection, and thus the two groups could not be compared directly. They overcame the problem by controlling for the factors using a sophisticated statistical technique (logistic regression). The analysis revealed that breast fed babies were protected against infection compared to their bottle fed compatriots. This type of analytical technique is described in the texts listed at the end of this chapter. What this example illustrates is the care which must be taken when using comparison groups.

Comparing with the General Community

Sometimes a convenient comparison group is unavailable. For example, during a follow-up of 513 patients with Crohn's disease, 102 were found to have died (25). As these patients were followed on average for 14.5 years some of them would be expected to have died, even if they did not have Crohn's disease. How can we decide if these patients are dying more quickly than healthy persons? The answer is to use the mortality rates of the general population to calculate the number of persons who would be expected to die. In the Crohn's disease study this method indicated that 51.8 deaths would be expected, suggesting that these patients were at twice the risk of dying as the general community. The calculation involved takes into account the age, sex and length of follow-up of each patient using some quite sophisticated statistical methods. Methods of analysis are described in texts by Breslow and Day (22), and Kahn (26).

Calculating Incidence Rates

Cohort studies can involve the calculation of an incidence rate. This is just a way of describing how frequently new cases of a disease occurred during the study. For example, if 23 cases of gastric cancer were diagnosed during a 10 year follow-up of 10 000 men, the result could be expressed as 23 cases per 10 000 men per 10 years. Incidence rates are often expressed per year rather than per 10 years. Using the assumption that, other things being equal, following 10 000 men for 10 years is the same as following 100 000 men for one year, the result can be re-expressed as 23 cases per 100 000 men per year. (This calculation illustrates the basic features of an incidence rate, although in practice it may be more complex: as men are followed over time some die and others are lost to follow-up. Allowance has to be made for these losses in the calculation of the incidence rate. Similarly, as men are followed up they get older and as many diseases, especially gastric cancer, increase in frequency with age, allowance has to be made for the ages of the men during the period of follow-up. There are standard methods for dealing with these issues and these are fully described in the books mentioned above.)

One study which expressed its findings as incidence rates was the Royal College of General Practitioners' study of mortality among users of oral contraceptives (27). This followed 23 000 women who had taken the pill and a similar number of controls who were matched by age and marital status. After five years' follow-up the death rate from diseases of the circulatory system was 26.8 per 100 000 women per year among oral contraceptive users, compared to 5.5 per 100 000 women per year among the controls. When results are expressed as incidence rates, they can be very easily summarised by the relative risk:

relative risk = incidence among the exposed/incidence among the non-exposed

In the oral contraceptive study, this becomes

relative risk = 26.8/5.5 = 4.9

This shows that the risk of diseases of the circulatory system was 4.9 times higher in the oral contraceptive users than among controls. The relative risk summarises the results of a cohort study in a single value. It is apparently simple to interpret, but a note of caution should be sounded about the meaning to be attached to it. Because two factors are associated, as for example the contraceptive pill and the risk of diseases of the circulatory system, does not mean that one causes the other. There may be other explanations. This potential pitfall, and others which can befall cohort studies, are discussed in the next section.

POTENTIAL PITFALLS

Like all methods in health services research, cohort studies suffer from a number of potential pitfalls. They are subject to bias. Bias is a general term for the types of process which can influence study results leading to misplaced interpretation. But in addition to this problem, cohort studies are sometimes subject to overenthusiastic interpretation. These two areas are discussed separately.

Sources of Bias

Cohort studies are subject to the forms of bias which are reviewed in detail in Chapter 15. But cohort studies are particularly prone to two forms of bias and these will be discussed here:

- selection bias
- losses to follow-up

Selection Bias

Cohort studies begin by selecting a sample of patients and are thus subject to the same types of selection bias as are surveys. It was pointed out in the chapter on surveys that the average severity of illness will increase from patients located in the community (many will have mild disease), through general practice to the hospital setting (where many will be severely ill). The outcome after follow-up will be strongly influenced by initial severity. This phenomenon was seen in a review of the long-term sequelae of childhood febrile seizures. It found a substantial range in the percentage of children with unfavourable sequelae (28). More detailed inspection showed that the population-based studies were consistent in their estimates of both febrile and non-febrile seizures, whereas clinic-based studies produced widely varying results. The authors reported: 'It is our basic conclusion that assessment of natural history from selected samples can produce misleading results.' The selection effect can be sufficiently strong to distort the findings completely. For example, a cohort study of survival of critically ill children in hospital made the surprising finding that the death rate was substantially higher in specialist units than in general hospitals (29). However, further investigation revealed that the children in the specialist units tended to be more seriously ill. When allowance was made for this in the analysis, children admitted to the specialist units were shown to have the better survival. It appeared that the general hospitals sent their most serious cases to the specialist centres.

Selection can also operate whenever patients can express a choice. For example, a cohort study of the effects on obstetric analgesia on the well-being of the babies compared women who chose pethidine, epidural bupivacaine, or no drug (30). However, the women opting for no analgesia were more likely to have had previous children, and had much shorter duration of labour and less frequently required oxytocin or forceps delivery. There can also be a difference in outcome between patients who comply well with therapy compared to those who do not. A study investigated survival by level of compliance of those taking a placebo drug, as part of a controlled clinical trial (31). It found that good compliers had a 40% reduction in mortality compared to poor compliers. When a cohort is being recruited, it is worth asking questions of the form: Where do these patients come from? Could there be a volunteer effect? Could there be selective referral? Answers to these questions could substantially affect the conclusions which can be drawn.

Losses to Follow-up

Losses to follow-up can introduce bias when those who drop out of the study differ from those who continue. This was investigated in a study of women's experience of postnatal care, because baseline data were available on those lost to follow-up (32). The study found those who were lost differed from those contacted in *'age, marital status, social class, and in the weight of their babies'*. Common reasons for loss to follow-up include: lack of interest in the study; moving home; death; or emigration. Omitting some of those who have died from a study can give an overoptimistic impression of the health of the study group. In contrast, omitting migrants, who might not migrate if they were ill, could lead to an overestimate of the amount of disease in the study group. The important point about losses to follow-up is that the bias can act in either direction.

Overenthusiastic Interpretation

The potential biases described above counsel caution when interpreting cohort studies. The findings of studies in medicine are not always what they seem. A classic study in epidemiology illustrates the dangers of interpreting an association between two variables as showing that one causes the other. When cholera was a health problem in London, it was found that the death rate from the disease fell with increasing height above the River Thames (33). This accorded with the theory of miasma, that disease was due to some contamination in the air. It was expected that contamination would decrease with altitude, and observation appeared to confirm this. Subsequent research showed that cholera was spread by contamination of drinking water with raw sewage. The findings could then be reinterpreted in terms of water purity. As stated previously, association does not mean causation.

Cohort studies should be treated with particular caution when deciding whether or not a treatment is effective. A number of review papers have pointed out that cohort studies give misleading results, often suggesting that treatment is more effective than it really is (34–36). In part the misplaced optimism can be explained by the natural history of the disease. Some patients would get better even without any intervention, and when included in a cohort study their improvements may be attributed to the treatment. However, there can be other explanations for treatments appearing effective. For example, a study compared open surgery versus percutaneous nephrolithotomy for the removal of kidney stones (37). The observation that nephrolithotomy had the higher success rate was found to be due to the kidney stones being on average smaller in this group of patients. When account was taken of this, open surgery appeared the better treatment. The problem is that in many circumstances it may not be obvious how the two groups differ, and the appropriate adjustment will never be made. The recognised valid method of assessing treatment efficacy, the randomised controlled clinical trial, is discussed in Chapter 8.

COMMENT AND FURTHER READING

Cohort studies can range in size and in the method and the length of follow-up. In many circumstances they can be simple to design and cheap to carry out. With a little care at the planning stage, major pitfalls can be avoided. Thus they are an ideal method for health care professionals to employ to answer the common question: What happens to these patients in the future? For example, in a follow-up study of patients with duodenal ulcer (23), a large effect was being sought: the question being asked was: *'Do a substantial number of patients remain free from* H. pylori *infection?'* Similarly, a study of the longer-term outcome of infantile hypertrophic pyloric stenosis was seeking only to determine whether adverse sequelae were rare: they were (38).

In some circumstances cohort studies will require very sophisticated statistical techniques for analysis. This can occur when subtle effects are being investigated. Special techniques will also be required when several different factors are likely to affect the outcome. In these circumstances advice should be sought from a statistician.

Books by Friedman (39), Lilienfeld and Lilienfeld (40) and Alderson (41) provide good introductory chapters to cohort studies. More advanced texts which describe in detail the design and the methods of analysis are by Breslow and Day (22), Rothman (42), Kahn (26) and Kleinbaum and colleagues (43). Guidelines for the critical analysis of published cohort studies are given in papers by the Department of Clinical Epidemiology and Biostatistics at McMaster University (44, 45) and by Laupacis and colleagues (46).

REFERENCES

1. Bilsland, D, Crombie, IK and Ferguson, J. The photosensitivity dermatitis and actinic reticuloid syndrome: no association with lymphoreticular malignancy. *British Journal of Dermatology* 1994; **131**: 209–14.

2. Möller, H, Knudsen, LB and Lynge, E. Risk of testicular cancer after vasectomy: cohort study of over 73000 men. *British Medical Journal* 1994; **309**: 295–9.

3. Jylhä, M. Ten-year change in the use of medical drugs among the elderly—a longitudinal study and cohort comparison. *Journal of Clinical Epidemiology* 1994; **47**(1): 69–79.

4. Hutton, JL, Cooke, T and Pharoah, POD. Life expectancy in children with cerebral palsy. *British Medical Journal* 1994; **309**: 431–5.

5. Cockerell, OC, Johnson, AL, Sander, JWAS, Hart, YM, Goodridge, DMG and Shorvon, SD. Mortality from epilepsy: results from a prospective population-based study. *Lancet* 1994; **344**: 918–21.

6. Milne, RIG. Assessment of care of children with sickle cell disease: implications for neonatal screening programmes. *British Medical Journal* 1990; **300**: 371–4.

7. Howie, PW, Forsyth, JS, Ogston, SA, Clark, A and Florey, CdV. Protective effect of breast feeding against infection. *British Medical Journal* 1990; **300**: 11–16.

8. Ratcliffe, F, Lawson, R and Millar, J. Day-case laparoscopy revisited: have post-operative morbidity and patient acceptance improved? *Health Trends* 1994; **26**(2): 47–9.

9. Crombie, IK, Brown, SV and Hamley, JG. Postmarketing drug surveillance by record linkage in Tayside. *Journal of Epidemiology and Community Health* 1984; **38**(3): 226–31.

10. Kind, P. Outcome measurement using hospital activity data: deaths after surgical procedures. *British Journal of Surgery* 1990; **77**: 1399–402.

11. Chambers, M and Clarke, A. Measuring readmission rates. *British Medical Journal* 1990; **301**: 1134–6.

12. Mukherjee, AK, Leck, I, Langley, FA and Ashcroft, C. The completeness and accuracy of health authority and cancer registry records according to a study of ovarian neoplasms. *Public Health* 1991; **105**: 69–78.

13. Pringle, M and Hobbs, R. Large computer databases in general practice [editorial]. *British Medical Journal* 1991; **302**: 741–2.

14. Pears, J, Alexander, V, Alexander, GF and Waugh, NR. Audit of the quality of hospital discharge data. *Health Bulletin* (Edinburgh) 1992; **50**(5): 356–61.

15. Wilson, APR, Weavill, C, Burridge, J and Kelsey, MC. The use of the wound

scoring method 'ASEPSIS' in postoperative wound surveillance. *Journal of Hospital Infection* 1990; **16**: 297–309.

16. de Haan, R, Limburg, M, van der Meulen, J and van den Bos, GAM. Use of health care services after stroke. *Quality in Health Care* 1993; **2**: 222–7.

17. Harrison, G, Mason, P, Glazebrook, C, Medley, I, Croudace, T and Docherty, S. Residence of incident cohort of psychotic patients after 13 years of follow up. *British Medical Journal* 1994; **308**: 813–16.

18. Newens, AJ, Forster, DP, Kay, DWK, Kirkup, W, Bates, D and Edwardson, J. Clinically diagnosed presenile dementia of the Alzheimer type in the Northern Health Region: ascertainment, prevalence, incidence and survival. *Psychological Medicine* 1993; **23**: 631–44.

19. Cutler, SJ, Schneiderman, MA and Greenhouse, SW. Some statistical considerations in the study of cancer in industry. *American Journal of Public Health* 1954; **44**: 1159–66.

20. Schlesselman, JJ. Sample size requirements in cohort and case-control studies of disease. *American Journal of Epidemiology* 1974; **99**(6): 381–4.

21. Lemeshow, S, Hosmer, DW Jr, Klar, J and Lwanga, SK. *Adequacy of Sample Size in Health Studies*. Chichester: John Wiley & Sons, 1990.

22. Breslow, NE and Day, NE. *Statistical Methods in Cancer Research. Volume II: The Design and Analysis of Cohort Studies.* Lyon: International Agency for Research on Cancer, 1987.

23. Forbes, GM, Glaser, ME, Cullen, DJE, *et al.* Duodenal ulcer treated with *Helicobacter pylori* eradication: seven-year follow-up. *Lancet* 1994; **343**: 258–60.

24. Baird, PA, Yee, IML and Sadovnick, AD. Population-based study of long-term outcomes after amniocentesis. *Lancet* 1994; **344**: 1134–6.

25. Prior, P, Gyde, S, Cooke, WT, Waterhouse, JAH and Allan, RN. Mortality in Crohn's disease. *Gastroenterology* 1981; **80**(2): 307–12.

26. Kahn, HA. *An Introduction to Epidemiologic Methods.* New York: Oxford University Press, 1983.

27. Beral, V. Mortality among oral-contraceptive users. Royal College of General Practitioners' Oral Contraception Study. *Lancet* 1977; **ii**: 727–31.

28. Ellenberg, JH and Nelson, KB. Sample selection and the natural history of disease. Studies of febrile seizures. *Journal of the American Medical Association* 1980; **243**(13): 1337–40.

29. Pollack, MM, Alexander, SR, Clarke, N, Ruttimann, UE, Tesselaar, HM and Bachulis, AC. Improved outcomes from tertiary center pediatric intensive care: a statewide comparison of tertiary and nontertiary care facilities. *Critical Care Medicine* 1991; **19**: 150–9.

30. Lieberman, BA, Rosenblatt, DB, Belsey, E, *et al.* The effects of maternally administered pethidine or epidural bupivacaine on the fetus and newborn. *British Journal of Obstetric Gynaecology* 1979; **86**: 598–606.

31. The Coronary Drug Project Research Group. Influence of adherence to treatment and response of cholesterol on mortality in the Coronary Drug Project. *New England Journal of Medicine* 1980; **303**(18): 1038–41.

32. Glazener, C, Abdalla, M, Russell, I and Templeton, A. Postnatal care: a survey of patients' experiences. *British Journal of Midwifery* 1993; **1**(2): 67–74.

33. Langmuir, AD. Epidemiology of airborne infection. *Bacteriological Reviews* 1961; **25**: 173–81.

34. Foulds, GA. Clinical research in psychiatry. *Journal of Mental Science* 1958; **104**(435): 259–65.

35. Chalmers, TC, Block, JB, Lee, S. Controlled studies in clinical cancer research. *New England Journal of Medicine* 1972; **287**(2): 75–8.
36. Gilbert, JP, McPeek, B, Mosteller, F. Statistics and ethics in surgery and anesthesia. *Science* 1977; **198**: 684–9.
37. Mays, N, Challah, S, Patel, S, *et al.* Clinical comparison of extracorporeal shock wave lithotripsy and percutaneous nephrolithotomy in treating renal calculi. *British Medical Journal* 1988; **297**: 253–8.
38. Zhang, A-L, Cass, DT, Dawson, KP and Cartmill, T. A medium term follow-up study of patients with hypertrophic pyloric stenosis. *Journal of Paediatrics and Child Health* 1994; **30**: 126–8.
39. Friedman, GD. *Primer of Epidemiology* 3rd edn. New York: McGraw-Hill, 1987.
40. Lilienfeld, AM and Lilienfeld, DE. *Foundations of Epidemiology* 2nd edn. New York: Oxford University Press, 1980.
41. Alderson, M. *An Introduction to Epidemiology* 2nd edn. London: Macmillan Press, 1983.
42. Rothman, KJ. *Modern Epidemiology*. Boston: Little, Brown, 1986.
43. Kleinbaum, DG, Kupper, LL and Morgenstern, H. *Epidemiologic Research. Principles and Quantitative Methods*. New York: Van Nostrand Reinhold, 1982.
44. Department of Clinical Epidemiology and Biostatistics MUHSC. How to read clinical journals: III. To learn the clinical course and prognosis of disease. *Canadian Medical Association Journal* 1981; **124**: 869–72.
45. Department of Clinical Epidemiology and Biostatistics MUHSC. How to read clinical journals: IV. To determine etiology or causation. *Canadian Medical Association Journal* 1981; **124**: 985–90.
46. Laupacis, A, Wells, G, Richardson, WS and Tugwell, P. Users' guides to the medical literature. V. How to use an article about prognosis. *Journal of the American Medical Association* 1994; **272**(3): 234–7.

Chapter 8

CLINICAL TRIALS

The effectiveness of health care can be assessed by comparing one form of care delivery against another. The idea of comparing treatments to see which is the better is not new. In his history of clinical trials, Bull (1) describes how James Lind in 1753 carried out a comparison of treatments for scurvy among sailors. Lind observed that *'the most sudden and visible good effects were perceived from the use of oranges and lemons'*. This chapter describes the ways in which the effectiveness of health care activities can be assessed, and outlines the requirements for the design of rigorous studies.

RANGE OF USES

The clinical trial is the recognised method for assessing the effectiveness of health care interventions. Clinical trials are often described in terms of drug therapy, but they can be used to assess any aspect of health care. Thus they have been used to assess:

- the contribution of psychosocial services to rehabilitation of intravenous drug users (2)
- the role of health visitors in preventing fractures in elderly people (3)
- the effects of aerobic exercise on the volume of breast milk produced by lactating women (4)
- the value of counselling in general practice (5)
- the efficacy of two days' compared with seven days' bed rest for acute low back pain (6)
- the effectiveness of geriatric rehabilitative care after fracture of the proximal femur in elderly women (7)
- the value of chiropractic manipulation in the treatment of low back pain (8)

These examples show that clinical trials can be used to investigate the overall effects of a care programme as well as the individual elements of that care. Clinical trials have also been widely used to investigate the impact of continuing medical education on the quality of clinical care (9), and to assess the impact of guidelines on clinical practice (10).

In short, clinical trials can be used to look at any aspect of health care delivery to answer the questions: Does it work? Does it lead to an improvement in patient care? The improvement may be measured in terms of the health of the patient; but it could also refer to the surgical skills of doctors, the efficiency of health care delivery or the well-being of bereaved relatives. There is often more than one way of organising and delivering health care. The clinical trial provides a means for determining which is the better alternative.

THE NEED FOR RIGOROUS STUDIES

Carrying out clinical trials can be a difficult business. There are many aspects of their design and execution which must be handled with great care. The difficulties which clinical trials present sometimes lead to suggestions that simpler alternative methods should be used to assess the benefits of health care interventions. Thus it is worth reviewing some examples which show the need for clinical trials and indicate the types of problem which can afflict other methods. Most of the examples involve an assessment of drug therapy, because this is the area of medicine in which trials have been most widely used. However, the points which they raise apply to all areas of health care.

Spontaneous Improvement

A recurring observation in medicine is that many patients show improvements in their condition irrespective of treatment. Infectious diseases, like colds and flu, are often self-limiting and the benefit of treatment may only be to reduce the duration of illness. For example, successful antibiotic therapy for respiratory infections may only shorten the duration of symptoms by two to three days (11). Other diseases, such as rheumatoid arthritis and multiple sclerosis, are characterised by periods of relapse or exacerbation followed by some improvement or even freedom from symptoms. The possibility of spontaneous changes in disease activity can make it difficult to assess the effects of a treatment. If the patient did improve this might be unrelated to therapy. Alternatively, a treated patient may have become a little worse but the doctor would not know whether, in the absence of therapy, the patient might not have become very much worse. The clinical trial provides a valid means of assessing therapies when there are spontaneous changes in disease state.

Not All Treatments Are Effective

Not all treatments have evidence to support their use: *'the history of medicine is richly endowed with therapies that were widely used and then shown to be ineffective or frankly toxic'* (12). One notable example was the use of supplemental oxygen in the early management of premature babies. The therapy was introduced in the United States in the 1940s because it was hoped that it would increase the chances of the infants surviving (13). In fact, a clinical trial conducted in 1953 showed that retrolental fibroplasia, a form of blindness, occurred in 23% of infants receiving routine oxygen. The practice of giving oxygen routinely was rapidly abandoned.

Concern about the number of potentially useless therapies for rheumatism led to the establishment of the Unproven Remedies Committee (14). The field of cancer therapy also provides examples of unproven treatments. In the 1970s and 1980s Laetrile (derived from apricot seeds) was fashionable, and more recently shark cartilage has become popular (15). There is no satisfactory evidence that these treatments are effective.

The Importance of Small Effects

Dramatic improvements in treatment are easy to demonstrate. For example, symptomatic rabies infection is always fatal, so that a few case reports of successful treatment would provide evidence to support a new therapy. Unfortunately, dramatic improvements in patient outcome are comparatively rare. Instead new developments usually offer small but clinically important advances. A good example of this is the treatment of childhood leukaemia, where a series of small advances have led to a substantial improvement in survival. This need to be able to detect modest improvements in outcome increases the need for rigorous study design.

The Limitations of Theory

In some instances there can be supportive evidence which suggests that a treatment ought to work. A good example of this is the cardiac arrhythmia suppression trial which was described in an editorial in the *New England Journal of Medicine* (12). There was good evidence that patients who had had a heart attack were at higher risk of dying if they had ventricular extrasystoles. There was also evidence that these extrasystoles could be suppressed by antiarrhythmic drugs. So it seemed reasonable that patients who had the extrasystoles would benefit from the antiarrhythmic drugs. Unfortunately it did not turn out this way. In the trial which was conducted 7.7% of patients given the drug died. In contrast, among the control group who were given a placebo (non-active tablet), only 3.0% of patients died. It appeared that the drug was causing rather than preventing sudden death.

Another graphic illustration of the limitations of theory is the radical mastectomy for breast cancer. The operation was proposed by Halstead in the late nineteenth century, because it was thought that breast cancer first spread locally and should therefore be treated by radical surgery. When patients continued to die, it was argued that the operation was not radical enough: *'this even went so far as to encourage surgeons in the 1920s to carry out forequarter amputations for locally advanced carcinoma of the breast'* (16). Clinical trials carried out since the 1950s demonstrated convincingly that *'radical treatment produces no benefit in surgery compared with the most conservative regimes'* (16). The general message is that treatments which should work in theory sometimes do not work in practice.

TYPES OF COMPARISON GROUPS

The key element in studies of the value of a new treatment is comparison. For example, breast shells have been used for more than 50 years to help pregnant women with inverted or non-protractile nipples prepare for breast feeding. One study found that 29% of women recommended to use the shells were breast feeding at six weeks after delivery (17). How can this result be interpreted? The answer is a comparison group (or control group) of women who had not used the shells. The study found that 50% of the control group were breast feeding at six weeks. One possible explanation for this is that emphasising the potential problems of breast feeding has a deterrent effect.

Comparison groups provide a yardstick against which treatments or health care interventions can be assessed. One misconception about clinical trials which can be quickly dismissed is that the control group is always given a placebo, i.e. a dummy treatment. This is not the case.

The control group is given the best available current treatment, and only if no effective treatment is available is a placebo used.

When making comparisons the two groups must be similar, so that any differences seen between them can be ascribed to the treatments each received. There are a number of comparison groups which could be used and these are reviewed below.

Comparisons Against Previously Treated Patients

A readily available comparison group are the patients who were seen in the recent past and received the conventional treatment. The hope is that by careful review of the case records it will be possible to select a set of patients who are similar to those receiving the new treatment. The patients from the past are referred to as historical controls, but their use is problematic. There is substantial evidence that studies which use them can be misleading; they *'tend to exaggerate the value of a new treatment'* (18). This was borne out in a review of studies of the treatment of colon cancer with 5-FU adjuvant (19). The two studies which used historical controls reported that the treatment was effective. However, when tested in five studies which used a more rigorous design, the treatment was shown to be of no value. Similar findings were made when reviews were conducted on treatments for other diseases ranging from cirrhosis with oesophageal varices to acute myocardial infarction (19).

A number of factors can conspire to make historical controls unsatisfactory. The types of patients seen may change over time because of changes in patterns of referral. Or there may have been changes in ancillary care which affect the recovery of patients. It can also be difficult to assess the outcome of treatment in historical cases, and it is unlikely that exactly the same criteria were used in the assessment of recent and historical cases. Historical controls are basically unreliable.

Concurrent Controls

It might be thought that many of the difficulties of historical controls could be avoided by using concurrent controls. These are patients who are seen at the same time but receive different therapy to that under investigation. The problem is that there will usually be good reasons why some patients did not receive the experimental treatment: they may have been under the care of another physician, or may have refused to consent to the new treatment, or there may have been clear indications that some other treatment was to be preferred. Whatever the reasons, it is likely that the clinical course of these patients would differ from those given the new treatment.

The problems of using concurrent controls are illustrated by the investigation of the survival of patients with breast cancer treated at the Bristol Cancer Help Centre (BCHC). This centre offers alternative treatments: a special diet, counselling and therapies designed to enhance quality of life. The survival of women attending the centre was compared against women with breast cancer who were treated conventionally at the Royal Marsden Hospital. Survival was found to be poorer among women attending the BCHC. This effect persisted when allowance was made for differences between the two groups of women at entry to the study (20). The findings provoked a controversy and led to further analyses being conducted. These took account of further differences between the two groups at entry. The difference in survival remained significantly poorer in the BCHC women, although the effect was smaller than first reported (21). Doubt remains about the benefits of the alternative therapy at BCHC, although it is likely that 'the study's results can be explained by the fact that women going to Bristol had more severe disease than control women' (22).

Perhaps the most disappointing feature of this affair is that the researchers who conducted the study had wished to employ à method which would have overcome the difficulties encountered—they were unable to do so because of objections from the BCHC. Their preferred method would have used randomised controls.

Randomised Controls

The problem with the control groups discussed above is that there can be systematic differences between those receiving the experimental treatment and those getting the comparison treatment. Even when they appear similar, doubt remains over all the unknown factors which might influence patient recovery. A fair assessment can only be made when 'treatments are compared under broadly similar circumstances' (23). In other words, the patients receiving one treatment should be broadly similar to those receiving the other. This can be achieved by recruiting a set of patients and then randomly allocating them to receive either the experimental treatment or the standard one. The result is that half the patients receive the new experimental treatment and the other half receive some other therapy. Randomisation can only be achieved by following a set procedure: 'random does not mean the same as haphazard: random allocation *in a clinical trial means that all patients have the same chance of receiving any particular treatment'* (24). When this is carried out the two groups should be similar in terms of important variables like age, sex and disease severity. The larger the number of patients recruited to the trial, the more likely that the two groups will be evenly balanced on all the factors which can influence patient outcome. The important point here is that we do not need to know what these factors are: randomising patients makes it very likely that the groups are similar. When the two groups are similar at the start of the study any difference which arises between them can be attributed to the effects of treatment.

DESIGN MATTERS

Clinical trials are carried out to a strict methodology. It is only too easy to design poor trials which yield inconclusive results. For example, a review of 23 trials of physiotherapy exercises for back pain found that the quality of the studies was so poor that *'no conclusion can be drawn about whether exercise therapy is better than other conservative treatments'* (25). There are several issues which need to be considered:

- definition of the patient group
- randomisation
- ethics
- outcome assessment
- patient follow-up
- blinding
- sample size

Definition of the Patient Group

The starting point for a clinical trial is a clear definition of the patients to be studied. This involves clarifying who is likely to benefit from treatment. Thus a study of bed rest for acute low back pain excluded patients for a variety of reasons, including those who were receiving steroids or anticoagulants, had pain located above T12, were seeking disability compensation, or had alcohol or drug abuse or a history of cancer. The reason for these exclusions was *'to assemble a group with uncomplicated mechanical back pain'* (6), presumably because the authors expected that the effects of treatment would be seen more clearly in this group.

Patients for whom there is a clear preference for one of the two treatments should also be excluded. This is why a study of the value of routine ultrasound screening in pregnancy excluded women who had had a previous perinatal loss, or had a history of diabetes, hypertension or kidney disease (26). These women would be given an ultrasound scan as part of normal clinical practice and thus could not be allocated to the non-screened group.

It is also important to exclude those for whom either of the proposed treatments is contraindicated. Thus in a study of chiropractic manipulation for low back pain, patients were excluded if they had major structural abnormalities visible on X-ray, or had osteopenia (8). Patients who have received one of the treatments previously are also usually excluded. Many such patients will have obtained little benefit from the therapy on the first occasion, so that including them might obscure a treatment effect.

The inclusion and exclusion criteria need to be constructed with some care, lest they result in an atypical group of patients being studied. This would limit the extent to which the findings can be generalised. Before undertaking any trial, attention should be given to whether the findings will be relevant to a broader group of patients.

Randomisation

In theory patients can be randomised to one of two groups by considering each patient in turn and tossing a coin: if it comes down heads the patient is allocated to one group, and to the other group if the coin is tails. A coin was used to assign treatments in a trial in 1931 of gold thiosulphate for pulmonary tuberculosis (23). But nowadays coins are seldom used. Instead the researcher can use the tables of random numbers printed in most statistics books. Alternatively, contact could be made with a statistician, who will probably use a computer to generate a convenient printout of randomisation codes. However the randomisation is carried out, it is essential that the details of it are recorded carefully so that when the results are analysed the patients can be correctly allocated to their treatment groups. The worst nightmare of researchers doing clinical trials is that the randomisation codes, indicating what treatment each patient received, become lost and the trial can never be analysed.

There are more sophisticated forms of randomisation which are used to make it even more likely that the two groups of patients are broadly similar. These are clearly described in a very good book by Pocock (18).

Ethics

All studies involving patients have ethical implications and these are discussed in Chapter 14. But clinical trials are a form of planned experiments on human beings, and they raise a number of special concerns. These are:

- withholding treatment
- modification to treatment
- informed consent

In essence, a clinical trial involves allowing chance rather than clinical judgement to decide which of two treatments a patient receives. In some circumstances the one treatment will be a new one which may offer a substantial therapeutic benefit. The possibility of gaining this benefit will be denied to half the patients recruited to the study. Can this be justified? The answer is a clear 'yes', provided certain conditions are met. First, it should be noted, as discussed above, that treatments which are new are not necessarily better. It is when this uncertainty exists that it becomes ethical to randomise patients to one or other treatment. Thus a clinical trial is ethical when, after careful review, *'the responsible physician is substantially uncertain as to which of the trial treatments would be most appropriate for this particular patient'* (27). When there are clinical grounds for preferring one option, the patient should not be entered into the trial but should be given the preferred option instead. Otherwise there is no ethical difficulty of randomly assigning patients to one or other group.

A second ethical concern is whether, once entered into the study, the patient can have the trial treatment stopped or modified in any way. The answer is similar to that governing entry to the trial; if there are good clinical grounds for thinking that therapy should be changed, then it should be changed. Patients should always be transferred from one therapy to the other, if the responsible physician is reasonably certain that this is warranted (27): *'individuals must never be denied clearly appropriate treatment, even if trial protocols are thereby disrupted'* (28).

Informed consent is the process of giving patients information about their disease and the treatments offered in the trial, so that they can decide whether or not they wish to take part. The issue was first raised in the early 1960s (29), but even in 1988 an eminent researcher pointed out that: *'Patients have until lately had little interest in or understanding of clinical trials. They are still mostly passive participants in trials, unwitting beneficiaries of the results, ignorant victims of the mistakes'* (30). For example, in a clinical trial designed to assess the side effects of oral contraceptives, some women were unknowingly given placebo tablets. Although these women were advised to use vaginal cream as well, *'six pregnancies occurred in the group receiving dummy pills'* (31). This practice has now changed. All participants must receive a thorough explanation of the nature of the study, and have to give consent in writing before they can be recruited to a trial.

Outcome Assessment

To be able to decide between alternative therapies, a formal method of evaluating the health of the patient is needed. In some circumstances the choice is straightforward. Thus in a study which compared methods of preventing fractures in elderly people, the natural outcome measure was the frequency with which fractures occurred (3). In other studies there may be a choice of outcome measure which could be used. The trial of the effect of exercise on breast milk of lactating women was concerned not just with the volume of milk produced, but with its composition (lipid, protein and lactose concentration and energy density) and the milk intake and body weight of the infants (4). It is recommended (18) that when there are several possible measures, one is nominated as the primary end point.

The choice of outcome assessment needs to be made with care. For example, in a trial of the management of hypertension one possible outcome would be the extent to which the treatment reduced blood pressure. But the important clinical question is not whether blood pressure is lowered, but whether the clinical consequences of hypertension, strokes and heart attacks, occur less frequently. Some patients may be mildly inconvenienced by raised blood pressure, but all would be concerned about suffering a stroke. Thus in its trial of anti-hypertensive agents, the Medical Research Council chose mortality and morbidity from strokes and coronary heart disease as primary endpoint measures (32).

It is not always clear which are the most clinically important measures. This will depend on the setting and purposes of the trial. For example, a review of the design issues of trials for patients with multiple sclerosis listed a number of candidates for outcome assessment, including the frequency of relapses, lower extremity function, upper extremity function, and a disability status score (33). Although the frequency of relapses might appear to be the most useful, the disability score was chosen because it is sensitive to disease progression, and because of a *'general consensus that a diminution in progression of the disease is much more important than a decrease in relapse rate'*.

Patient Follow-up

Clinical trials are much simpler to carry out if the outcome assessment is made shortly after randomisation. Trials in which patients are followed up over extended periods of time run the risk of losing contact with patients. The MRC hypertension trial followed patients for just over five years. During this time contact was lost with 25% of those recruited. Losses on this scale could threaten the validity of the study. Fortunately for the MRC study, it was possible to trace the missing patients through the NHS central register at Southport (see Chapter 7 for details), so that useful results were obtained. Those who disappear from view cause concern because they may be different to those who remain in contact. They could either be sicker than average, disappearing because of admission to other hospitals or death. Or they could be healthier than average, disappearing because they have moved house or emigrated. It is even possible that those disappearing from one treatment group are mainly healthy, whereas those disappearing from the other group are mainly sick. Whatever way it works out, substantial losses to follow-up can introduce bias and negate the value of a study.

Blinding

Like any other research method, clinical trials are subject to bias. In clinical trials the bias can come in unusual guises, affecting the patient, the researcher or even the statistician analysing the data. This set of biases is prevented using a set of techniques collectively called blinding.

When patients are given a treatment which they believe to be beneficial, they often show substantial improvement even if they have been given the placebo therapy. This phenomenon, the placebo response, has been seen in many different clinical settings. For example, in a trial of the effect of a hair restorer on male baldness, the treated group had an average increase of 133 hairs on a five centimetre square, but the control group also had a substantial average increase of 109 hairs (34). About 40% of both groups reported being satisfied with the cosmetic effect of the new hair growth. In this study none of the patients knew which treatment they were receiving, although many may have hoped it was the active one. If those on the placebo had been told that their treatment was an ineffective one, many fewer might have experienced the apparent benefit. In contrast, if the group receiving the active treatment had known this, their wish for hair regrowth might have augmented their response. For ethical reasons the patients must be told that they are in a trial, and know what the different treatments are. But to prevent the placebo effect from obscuring the true response to treatment, patients are not told which treatment they are to receive. This type of study is described as being single blind.

A double-blind trial is one in which *'neither the patient nor those responsible for his care and evaluation know which treatment he is receiving'* (18). Knowing which treatment patients receive could influence clinical judgement, especially when assessing the extent to which the patients have responded to therapy. A study of the treatment of multiple sclerosis investigated this problem by having all patients assessed by two neurologists, one who knew the treatment details and one who did not (35). Although the blinded assessment showed no effect of treatment, the assessments by the neurologist who knew the treatment groups produced an apparent treatment effect which was statistically significant. The authors concluded: *'physician blinding prevented an erroneous conclusion about treatment efficacy'*.

Statisticians are just as susceptible to bias as anyone else. Thus when there are several outcome measures which could be investigated, and lots of subgroups to be explored, the desire to find some sort of treatment effect could lead to overenthusiastic data interpretation. This will not happen if the statistician is blinded to the nature of the treatment groups, referring to them only as treatment I and treatment II. This is termed triple blinding.

Sample Size

Many clinical trials are simply not large enough. One clinician pointed out: *'it is worrying to observe such a profusion of clinical trials in dermatology which are too small to answer the questions being posed'* (36). The shortfall in numbers is not limited to dermatology. A review of trials of infertility treatment (37) found that the average study contained 96 patients, whereas over ten times that number would be needed to have a reasonable chance of detecting a successful treatment. The inadequacy of sample sizes has also been criticised in reviews of trials of antibiotics for acute bronchitis (38), and in the pharmacotherapy of sexual offenders (39).

The reason for this concern with size is that trials which are small will often fail to detect a treatment effect which would be clinically important. Unfortunately, *'clinical trials are not as sensitive as one would suppose to quite substantial differences between treatments, because random*

Table 8.1 Sample sizes required to detect clinically worthwhile treatment effects as being statistically significant*

% of control group showing an improvement	Additional benefit caused by treatment	Total number of patients required for	
		80% chance of detecting an effect	90% chance of detecting an effect
50%	5%	3208	4268
	10%	814	1076
	20%	206	268
	30%	90	114
70%	5%	2580	3428
	10%	626	824
	20%	142	184

* taking p<0.05 as the level of statistical significance

differences between different groups of patients are so much larger than one might expect' (28). These differences can obscure the effects of the therapy under test. Trials which are very small spurn an opportunity to detect clinically worthwhile treatments. They are also unethical, because patients are being entered into studies which are unlikely to provide useful information.

An indication of the size of trials which may be required is shown in Table 8.1. Because the play of chance is always with us, there is never a guarantee that a particular study will detect a benefit of therapy even if it exists. The best one can do is to specify what chance a study has of finding an effect of a given size. Thus the table presents the overall number of patients for the two treatment groups combined for two different scenarios: one in which the study has an 80% chance of detecting an effect, and one in which it has a 90% chance of doing so.

To illustrate the use of the table, consider a study in which 70% of patients with acute low back pain would be expected to recover spontaneously within four weeks. Suppose a pain management programme increased the proportion who recovered by 10% so that 80% now recover. The second last column of the table shows that it would require a study with 626 patients to detect an improvement of this size as being statistically significant. Even then we cannot be certain that the effect will be detected—only 80% sure. The calculation of the required sample size depends on three factors: how large the effect of treatment is likely to be; the level of statistical significance to be used; and how likely it is that a particular study will detect a real treatment difference. In this example the treatment effect was 10%, the significance level was p<0.05, and there was an 80% chance of detecting the effect. The table shows that a few hundred patients would be required to detect even quite large treatment effects. Much larger numbers would be required to detect smaller but worthwhile treatment effects.

Before beginning a clinical trial, the required sample size should be calculated to determine whether it is worth proceeding. The technical details of how sample size calculations are performed are given in books by Pocock (18) and Lemeshow and colleagues (40). Papers by Boag and colleagues (41), Altman (42) and Miller and Homan (43) present graphical aids to help select the appropriate sample size. However, as always, it would be easier to contact a local friendly statistician for advice.

ANALYSIS AND INTERPRETATION

In some clinical trials the analysis can be comparatively straightforward. The trial of the effect of health visitors on fractures in the elderly simply compared the proportion of fractures in the intervention group (5%) with the proportion in the control group (4%). This study was easy to analyse because the results of treatment could be expressed as a proportion. The analysis is also straightforward when the results can be expressed as an average (arithmetic mean). Thus the study of alopecia compared the average number of hairs in a five centimetre area on the heads of those receiving the hair restorer against the same measure in those not receiving it (34).

Although clinical trials can be simple to analyse, there are circumstances which can call for more sophisticated statistical techniques or for care in the interpretation of findings. Problems can arise in a number of areas:

- adjustment for group differences
- subgroup analyses
- losses to follow-up
- interpretation of negative studies

Adjustment for Group Differences

The analysis can become complex when the groups being compared are not well balanced on factors which could influence patient outcome. In the MRC hypertension study, diastolic blood pressure, sex, age and ECG changes were important predictors of mortality. Thus in the analysis allowance was made for these effects to enable the result of treatment to be seen. This sophisticated analysis is described in most good books, such as those listed at the end of Chapter 15.

Subgroup Analyses

In many clinical trials it is possible to subdivide patients by factors like age, sex, severity of disease, time since disease onset and many others. There may be theoretical reasons why some of these subgroups should benefit more from treatment than others. The analysis would then be extended from looking at all patients combined, to looking at selected subsets. This approach runs into trouble when large numbers of different subgroups are explored. It rapidly becomes almost certain that spuriously significant treatment effects will be observed. This will occur even when overall there is no difference between the two treatments being compared. To protect against misleading findings, it is best to specify in advance the few subgroups to be analysed.

Losses to Follow-up

Patients may leave a trial because they withdraw consent. Other patients may receive a treatment quite different to that to which they were allocated. This can occur when the physician responsible decides that it is in the patients' best interests to change therapy. Whatever the reasons patients come to leave a trial, every effort must be made to include them in the final analysis in the group to which they were first allocated. The practice of including all the patients in the analysis is called an *'intention to treat analysis'*. It is followed because of concerns that the reasons for patients leaving the trial may be related to the particular treatment they received. To take a somewhat extreme example, suppose that a treatment had no beneficial effect but instead caused unpleasant side effects in the most seriously ill patients. This could induce many of these patients to withdraw from the study. Those remaining would on average be much healthier than those in the comparison group (because the seriously ill would have no reason to withdraw from this group). In consequence the treatment would appear to be effective, although this result would only be due to the selective loss of seriously ill patients from one group. There are a number of different ways in which selective loss of patients can introduce bias into a study. The intention to treat analysis prevents any of these from occurring. This practice may dilute the size of effect which is detected, but it is nonetheless preferred to the possibility of introducing bias.

Interpretation of Negative Studies

Negative findings can present some difficulty for the interpretation of clinical trials. The trouble is that they could arise either because there was no difference between the treatments or because the study was too small to detect a difference. In general, unless the trial was very large indeed, it should not be assumed that there was no difference between the treatments. The section on sample size showed that large numbers of patients would often be needed to detect even quite sizable differences. To show that treatments are virtually equivalent requires very much larger studies (44). The question then is not of whether there was an effect of treatment, but of what size of effect is compatible with the study findings. If there was a negative finding, look first to see how large the study was.

PITFALLS

Pitfalls in clinical trials occur when insufficient attention has been paid to the design of the study, or to the analysis and interpretation of the results. Although these have been covered in the previous sections, it is worth listing together the main pitfalls. These are:

- poorly defined patient group
- failed randomisation
- inadequate sample size
- poor outcome measure
- poor blinding
- failure to comply with therapy
- patients lost to follow-up
- subgroup analyses

COMMENTS AND FURTHER READING

Clinical trials can be designed to be quick and simple to run and to produce results which are easily interpreted. For example, a study was carried out to determine whether patients responded better to a letter signed by their own general practitioner, or one sent directly from a research unit (45). The study involved little more than carrying out two postal surveys, with patients being randomly assigned to be in one or the other. The measure of outcome was whether or not the patients replied to the letter, with more patients responding to the letters from their GP. This study illustrates the three features which make clinical trials easy to conduct:

- patient group easily obtained
- short follow-up
- simple outcome measures

An easily obtained patient group is one where the inclusion and exclusion criteria are simply defined, and the patients are readily available. The benefit of a short follow-up is that it reduces the opportunities for patients to become lost. Simple outcome measures are those which involve counting easily observed events, such as responding to a letter.

In some circumstances clinical trials inevitably become complex. This can occur when there are insufficient patients at a single centre so that several centres have to become involved. Recruiting patients over extended periods as they gradually present at clinic also adds greatly to the difficulties of running a trial. Sometimes the outcome measure involves repeated assessments. For example, in the trial of chiropractic manipulation of low back pain, patient disability was assessed at weekly intervals for six weeks, at six months, and at one and two years (8). The resources needed for trials such as this will often be beyond those of individual researchers (the chiropractic trial received support from four separate funding bodies). Unless the researcher is experienced at running clinical trials and in obtaining external funding to meet the resource costs, these trials are best avoided.

Papers by Altman (46) and Pocock (47) provide a general introduction to clinical trials, and one by Warlow describes the complexities of multi-centre studies (48). An excellent guide to the presentation of the results from a clinical trial is given by Hampton (49). In his book on statistics, Altman (50) describes the design, analysis and interpretation of trials. But the best single source of information and advice on clinical trials is the book by Pocock (18).

REFERENCES

1. Bull, JP. The historical development of clinical therapeutic trials. *Journal of Chronic Diseases* 1959; **10**(3): 218–48.
2. McLellan, AT, Arndt, IO, Metzger, DS, Woody, GE and O'Brien, CP. The effects of psychosocial services in substance abuse treatment. *Journal of the American Medical Association* 1993; **269**(15): 1953–9.
3. Vetter, NJ, Lewis, PA and Ford, D. Can health visitors prevent fractures in elderly people? *British Medical Journal* 1992; **304**: 888–90.
4. Dewey, KG, Lovelady, CA, Nommsen-Rivers, LA, McCrory, MA and

Lönnerdal, B. A randomized study of the effects of aerobic exercise by lactating women on breast-milk volume and composition. *New England Journal of Medicine* 1994; **330**(7): 449–53.

5. King, M, Broster, G, Lloyd, M and Horder, J. Controlled trials in the evaluation of counselling in general practice. *British Journal of General Practice* 1994; **44**: 229–32.

6. Deyo, RA, Diehl, AK and Rosenthal, M. How many days of bed rest for acute low back pain? A randomized clinical trial. *New England Journal of Medicine* 1986; **315**(17): 1064–70.

7. Kennie, DC, Reid, J, Richardson, IR, Kiamari, AA and Kelt, C. Effectiveness of geriatric rehabilitative care after fractures of the proximal femur in elderly women: a randomised clinical trial. *British Medical Journal* 1988; **297**: 1083–6.

8. Meade, TW, Dyer, S, Browne, W, Townsend, J and Frank, AO. Low back pain of mechanical origin: randomised comparison of chiropractic and hospital outpatient treatment. *British Medical Journal* 1990; **300**: 1431–7.

9. Davis, DA, Thomson, MA, Oxman, AD and Haynes, RB. Evidence for the effectiveness of CME. A review of 50 randomized controlled trials. *Journal of the American Medical Association* 1992; **268**(9): 1111–17.

10. Weingarten, SR, Riedinger, MS, Conner, L, *et al*. Practice guidelines and reminders to reduce duration of hospital stay for patients with chest pain. *Annals of Internal Medicine* 1994; **120**(4): 257–63.

11. Davey, PG, Malek, MM and Parker, SE. Pharmacoeconomics of antibacterial treatment. *PharmacoEconomics* 1992; **1**(6): 409–37.

12. Passamani, E. Clinical trials—are they ethical? *New England Journal of Medicine* 1991; **324**(22): 1589–92.

13. Silverman, WA. The lesson of retrolental fibroplasia. *Scientific American* 1977; **236**: 100–107.

14. Lockshin, MD. The Unproven Remedies Committee. *Arthritis and Rheumatism* 1981; **24**(9): 1188–90.

15. Lowenthal, RM. On eye of newt and bone of shark. The dangers of promoting alternative cancer treatments [editorial]. *Medical Journal of Australia* 1994; **160**: 323–4.

16. Baum, M. Scientific empiricism and clinical medicine: a discussion paper. *Journal of the Royal Society of Medicine* 1981; **74**: 504–9.

17. Alexander, JM, Grant, AM, Campbell, MJ. Randomised controlled trial of breast shells and Hoffman's exercises for inverted and non-protractile nipples. *British Medical Journal* 1992; **304**: 1030–2.

18. Pocock, SJ. *Clinical Trials: A Practical Approach*. Chichester: John Wiley & Sons, 1983.

19. Sacks, H, Chalmers, TC, Smith, H Jr. Randomized versus historical controls for clinical trials. *American Journal of Medicine* 1982; **72**: 233–40.

20. Bagenal, FS, Easton, DF, Harris, E, Chilvers, CED and McElwain, TJ. Survival of patients with breast cancer attending Bristol Cancer Help Centre. *Lancet* 1990; **336**: 606–10.

21. Chilvers, CED, Easton, DF, Bagenal, FS, Harris, E and McElwain, TJ. Bristol Cancer Help Centre [letter]. *Lancet* 1990; **336**: 1186–8.

22. Bodmer, W. Bristol Cancer Help Centre [letter]. *Lancet* 1990; **336**: 1188.

23. Armitage, P. The role of randomization in clinical trials. *Statistics in Medicine* 1982; **1**: 345–52.

24. Altman, DG. Randomisation [editorial]. *British Medical Journal* 1991; **302**: 1481–2.

25. Koes, BW, Bouter, LM, Beckerman, H, van der Heijden, GJMG and Knipschild, PG. Physiotherapy exercises and back pain: a blinded review. *British Medical Journal* 1991; **302**: 1572–6.

26. Waldenström, U, Axelsson, O, Nilsson, S, *et al*. Effects of routine one-stage ultrasound screening in pregnancy: a randomised controlled trial. *Lancet* 1988; **ii**: 585–8.

27. Collins, R, Doll, R and Peto, R. Ethics of clinical trials. In: Williams, CJ, ed. *Introducing New Treatments for Cancer: Practical, Ethical and Legal Problems.* Chichester: John Wiley & Sons, 1992: 49–65.

28. Peto, R, Pike, MC, Armitage, P, *et al*. Design and analysis of randomized clinical trials requiring prolonged observation of each patient. I. Introduction and design. *British Journal of Cancer* 1976; **34**: 585–612.

29. Foster, CG. Research ethics committees in Britain. In: Williams, CJ, ed. *Introducing New Treatments for Cancer: Practical, Ethical and Legal Problems.* Chichester: John Wiley & Sons, 1992: 91–102.

30. Herxheimer, A. The rights of the patient in clinical research. *Lancet* 1988; **ii**: 1128–30.

31. Controlled trials: planned deception? [editorial]. *Lancet* 1979; **i**: 534–5.

32. MRC Working Party. Medical Research Council trial of treatment of hypertension in older adults: principal results. *British Medical Journal* 1992; **304**: 405–12.

33. Weiss, W and Stadlan, EM. Design and statistical issues related to testing experimental therapy in multiple sclerosis. In: Rudick, RA and Goodkin, DE, eds. *Treatment of Multiple Sclerosis: Trial Design, Results, and Future Perspectives.* London: Springer-Verlag, 1992: 91–122.

34. Kessels, AGH, Cardynaals, RLLM, Borger, RLL, *et al*. The effectiveness of the hair-restorer "Dabao"® in males with alopecia androgenetica. A clinical experiment. *Journal of Clinical Epidemiology* 1991; **44**(4/5): 439–47.

35. Noseworthy, JH, Ebers, GC, Vandervoort, MK, Farquhar, RE, Yetisir, E and Roberts, R. The impact of blinding on the results of a randomized, placebo-controlled multiple sclerosis clinical trial. *Neurology* 1994; **44**(1): 16–20.

36. Williams, HC and Seed, P. Inadequate size of "negative" clinical trials in dermatology. *British Journal of Dermatology* 1993; **128**(3): 317–26.

37. Vandekerckhove, P, O'Donovan, PA, Lilford, RJ and Harada, TW. Infertility treatment: from cookery to science. The epidemiology of randomised controlled trials. *British Journal of Obstetrics and Gynaecology* 1993; **100**(11): 1005–36.

38. Orr, PH, Scherer, K, Macdonald, A and Moffatt, ME. Randomized placebo-controlled trials of antibiotics for acute bronchitis: a critical review of the literature. *Journal of Family Practitioners* 1993; **36**(5): 507–12.

39. Richer, M, Crismon, ML. Pharmacotherapy of sexual offenders. *Annals of Pharmacotherapy* 1993; **27**(3): 316–20.

40. Lemeshow, S, Hosmer, DW Jr, Klar, J and Lwanga, SK. *Adequacy of Sample Size in Health Studies.* Chichester: John Wiley & Sons, 1990.

41. Boag, JW, Haybittle, JL, Fowler, JF and Emery, EW. The number of patients required in a clinical trial. *British Journal of Radiology* 1971; **44**(518): 122–5.

42. Altman, DG. Statistics and ethics in medical research. III How large a sample? *British Medical Journal* 1980; **281**: 1336–8.

43. Miller, DK and Homan, SM. Graphical aid for determining power of clinical trials involving two groups. *British Medical Journal* 1988; **297**: 672–6.

44. Makuch, RW and Johnson, MF. Some issues in the design and interpretation of "negative" clinical studies. *Archives of Internal Medicine* 1986; **146**: 986–9.

45. Smith, WCS, Crombie, IK, Campion, PD and Knox, JDE. Comparison of response rates to a postal questionnaire from a general practice and a research unit. *British Medical Journal* 1985; **291**: 1483–5.

46. Altman, DG. Statistics and ethics in medical research: study design. *British Medical Journal* 1980; **281**: 1267–9.

47. Pocock, SJ. Current issues in the design and interpretation of clinical trials. *British Medical Journal* 1985; **290**: 39–42.

48. Warlow, C. Organise a multicentre trial. *British Medical Journal* 1990; **300**: 180–3.

49. Hampton, JR. Presentation and analysis of the results of clinical trials in cardiovascular disease. *British Medical Journal* 1981; **282**: 1371–3.

50. Altman, DG. *Practical Statistics for Medical Research*. London: Chapman and Hall, 1991.

Chapter 9

CASE-CONTROL STUDIES

Studies which investigate selected samples of cases can sometimes be difficult to interpret. For example, if a study showed that 76% of men who had had a heart attack drank alcohol, it would be difficult to decide whether alcohol increased the risk of an attack. We would also need to know about the alcohol consumption of men who had not had a heart attack. These men would form a comparison or control group. If alcohol was associated with heart attacks, it should be more commonly consumed by those who had an attack than by the controls. A study which investigated this found that 82% of these controls consumed alcohol compared to 76% of heart attack patients (1). Alcohol consumption was less common in the cases. The authors concluded that far from causing heart disease, alcohol might protect against it. (The finding that moderate consumption is protective has been confirmed in a number of other studies (2).)

The alcohol and heart disease study is an example of a case-control study. The essence of case-control studies is that they provide a comparison group to assist the interpretation of findings. As with the other research methods, case-control studies follow a rigorous methodology. But they are much more prone to methodological problems, and their findings have to be interpreted with some care. This chapter reviews the range of uses of case-control studies, outlines the major features of study design, and highlights the problems confronting this method.

RANGE OF USES

The case-control approach can be used to assess the quality of care which has been given. Thus when Gaffney and colleagues were interested in the relationship between the quality of care during labour and delivery and the occurrence of cerebral palsy, they used a case-control study (3). The study found that poor care was associated with occurrence of cerebral palsy in only a small proportion of cases.

Case-control studies have also been used to investigate the attitudes and beliefs of users and non-users of preventive health care. For example, Orbell and colleagues (4) were concerned about women who did not attend for screening for cervical cancer, and investigated the reasons for this using a case-control study. The cases were all women aged 20–65 years (i.e. the age range at which screening is offered) who were recorded on a computer system as never having had a cervical smear. Controls were women who had had a smear within the previous three years. They found that it was anticipation of the embarrassment and pain of the smear, combined with a fear of a positive result being obtained, which deterred many of these women from attending.

A common use of case-control studies is to investigate factors which predict why some individuals experience an event and others do not. This method was used in this way to determine the causes of an outbreak of acute illness and death in a haemodialysis unit (5). Patients who became acutely ill were compared with patients attending the same unit who did not become ill. The outbreak was traced to defects in a temporary deionisation unit which resulted in some patients receiving fluoride intoxication. The case-control method has also been used to determine why some women have premature rupture of the amniotic membrane (6). The authors of the report hoped that the findings of an association of premature rupture with urinogenital infection would *'help physicians develop health care delivery strategies to identify and counsel patients at risk of preterm premature rupture of membranes'*.

Case-control studies are conventionally described where the cases are individuals who have a disease, and the controls are a suitable group of persons who do not have the disease. However, this is an unnecessarily restrictive view of the method. By using different definitions of cases, it is possible to extend the range of uses of case-control studies. For example, they could be used to investigate:

* why some patients respond well to therapy while others do not (cases would be those who did not respond and controls a similar set of patients who had responded);
* why only some medical students present for vaccination against hepatitis B;
* why some patients develop postoperative complications (the cases) and others undergoing the same operation do not (the controls). In this example both cases and controls have a disease (which is the reason for their surgery). It is the experience of postoperative complications which identifies the cases.

Thus being a case need not just mean having a disease. Cases have some defining characteristic: they may have suffered some adverse event, such as wound infection or emergency reoperation; or some event may not have happened, such as vaccination or screening for cervical cancer. In general case-control studies can be used to investigate patients or other individuals, or even pieces of equipment; the feature of cases is that they have some characteristic of interest.

Advantages of Case-control Studies

Case-control studies can be used in a variety of clinical settings to investigate a broad range of topics. One advantage of this method is that several potential differences between cases and controls can be examined within a single study. For example, the study of premature rupture of the amniotic membrane investigated several different types of infection (intra-amniotic, urinary tract, cervical gonococcal, cervical chlamydial) as well as exposure to cigarette smoke, previous rupture of membranes and antepartum bleeding (6).

Case-control studies are also ideally suited for investigating rare events. This is why the method was used to investigate rare diseases such as cerebral palsy. Focusing on the cases, and a suitable control group, means that data only have to be gathered on a relatively small number of individuals. This contrasts with using cohort studies to investigate rare events. Here data would have to be collected on a large number of individuals, to ensure that some cases would be included in the study. In consequence the study would be expensive to carry out and a large proportion of the data collected would be unnecessary. Case-control studies are usually smaller and cheaper.

DESIGN MATTERS

In principle case-control studies are quite straightforward to carry out, involving five activities:

* identify cases
* identify controls
* decide about matching
* estimate sample size
* collect data

Identify Cases

Cases are identified because they have a particular disease (e.g. cerebral palsy) or because they have some other defining characteristic (e.g. do not use a preventive health care service). Recruiting cases raises similar issues of representativeness that were encountered in drawing samples. The concern is to avoid an atypical set of cases. Thus in the study of cerebral palsy and intrapartum care (3), the cases were all children born with cerebral palsy in Oxford between 1984 and 1987 (with the additional requirements that the children were singletons, with a gestation of 37 weeks or more, and that there were no congenital anomalies and no postnatal causes of the cerebral palsy). Including all available cases limits the possible bias which could be introduced by including only selected infants. The exclusions were imposed to prevent other factors obscuring the association of interest; thus preterm and multiple pregnancy babies were excluded because they are already at increased risk of cerebral palsy for reasons unconnected with the quality of care.

Cases can be obtained from many different settings, from the community through general practice to the hospital. The same sources of cases that were used in surveys (see Table 6.2 in Chapter 6) can also be used to identify cases for case-control studies. It is worth noting again that the characteristics of patients will vary across settings, with relatively fewer severe cases in the community but many more of them in specialist hospitals. Thus the setting from which the cases are identified can influence the findings. A study of the factors associated with childhood accidents used different but overlapping sources of cases: all those who had an accident which required medical attention; and those whose accident was sufficiently serious to require hospital admission (7). The community cases were associated with young maternal age and area of residence, whereas the hospital cases were associated with young maternal age, large family and the loss or replacement of a natural parent (but not area of residence). The authors of the report concluded that there might be different subsets of children who have accidents.

When there is more than one source of cases, it is worth spending some time identifying which is the best. In this context best is a combination of ease of access and the types of cases which are likely to be obtained. There is no need for cases to be representative of all cases in the general population. What is important is that the members of the control group are selected in a similar way. Thus if the cases are identified as inpatients in a particular hospital, then controls should be selected from the same hospital. Similarly, if the cases were identified through a general practitioner, controls should also be selected from the GP's list. The only reservation to this argument is that it would be unhelpful to select cases which were so unusual that findings from the study cannot be widely applied. Some attention needs to be given to the questions: 'What are my cases like? To what extent can I generalise the findings to other types of cases?'

Identify Controls

The control group is chosen to be as similar to the cases as possible, except that its members do not have the disease or defining characteristic of the cases. In the cerebral palsy example (3), controls were selected from the hospital delivery book as being born immediately before each case (again with the requirements for singleton birth at 37 weeks' gestation or more, and with no congenital anomalies). Thus the controls were selected in the same way as cases, but with the proviso that they did not have cerebral palsy.

In general, if the cases were selected from a particular setting, say hospital inpatients, the controls should be selected from the same setting. Thus a study of the association between psychosocial factors and rheumatoid arthritis in the Lebanon used cases from hospital inpatients, outpatient departments and private clinics (8). Controls were obtained from the same institutions and matched to the cases by sex and age (within two years). The authors found that life-events were associated with an increased risk of arthritis, although the importance of psycho-social factors could be difficult to assess because the study was conducted during a war.

In some circumstances it may be appropriate to select controls from the general community. This was the approach adopted in a study of factors which influenced the likelihood of injury or death during a tornado (9). The locations of the victims at the time of injury was compared with the locations of members of the community who escaped injury. Injuries were found to occur to people who attempted to drive their cars out of the storm's path. Community controls should be chosen by first asking where the cases come from, then selecting controls to come from the same locality.

Many case-control studies select one control for each case. However, there is no theoretical requirement to have exactly the same number of cases and controls. When cases are easy to obtain, it is best to have an equal number of cases and controls. But when cases are difficult to find, if there are only 50 or 100 available, then equality may not be such a good thing. Instead, it can be useful to have two or three controls for every case. Increasing the number of controls increases the power of the study, making it more likely that an effect will be detected (should one exist). Thus a high power can be maintained when the number of cases is smaller than would have been wanted. Having more than one control per case increases the workload, but this can be worthwhile if there are few cases. However, there is little additional benefit in having more than four controls per case, so that the extra workload in obtaining them is unlikely to be justified.

Decide about Matching

There is one type of case-control study where the number of cases is exactly equal to the number of controls. This occurs when the cases are individually matched to the controls on factors like gender, age (say, to within one year), or marital status. The main reason for matching is to eliminate bias: it makes sure that cases and controls are similar for the matched factors (and any factors closely associated with the matching ones). Matching can also increase the power of a study, making it easier to detect what is going on.

But the gains of matching are only achieved at a price. The process of matching means that the straightforward analysis (described below) is no longer appropriate. Instead, more sophisticated statistical methods have to be used. These techniques are fully described in the book by Schlesselman (10).

Estimate Sample Size

A feature of case-control studies which is commonly emphasised is that they require smaller numbers than other methods. This may be true, but all too often it proves difficult to get as many cases as desired. Studies which have reported positive findings seldom contain fewer than 50 cases. Many case-control studies have 200–400 cases and some have analysed over 1000 cases. More details on this are given in Table 9.1, which shows the number of cases which would be required to have a reasonable chance of detecting a difference between cases and controls. Suppose in a study of cerebral palsy 20% of the cases had experienced some deficiency in care, such as an extended delay in responding to extreme distress. If only 10% of the controls experienced a delay, then a

Table 9.1 Sample sizes for case-control studies: number of cases required to have a reasonable chance* of detecting a difference between the cases and controls

Cases with factor being studied (%)	Controls with factor being studied (%)	No. of cases required (NB an equal no. of controls will be needed)
	10	219
	15	945
	25	1133
20	30	313
	35	151
	40	91
	40	407
	45	1604
	55	1604
50	60	407
	65	182
	70	103

*Technical note: reasonable chance corresponds to a significance level of 5% and a power of 80%

study with 219 cases (and an equal number of controls) would be needed to show a difference between cases and controls. (These estimates are fictitious but not unreasonable.) In general, Table 9.1 shows that small differences between cases and controls will require very large studies.

This section on sample sizes only gives a very rough guide to the size of study which might be necessary. In practice, a formal sample size calculation would have to be carried out. Many researchers find it better to ask a statistician to perform the necessary calculations, but those who wish to try for themselves will find useful advice in the paper by Schlesselman (11) and the books by Schlesselman (10) and Lemeshow and colleagues (12).

Collect Data

As with surveys, data on cases and controls are usually collected by interview or through self-completed questionnaires. The issues of data collection are described in Chapter 13. But some aspects are particularly important for case-control studies:

- limit the data collected
- standardise collection techniques
- use blinding

One of the features of case-control studies is that they can easily explore many possible differences between cases and controls. This can lead researchers into the temptation of collecting excessive amounts of data. This should be resisted. The items to be collected should be clarified when the research question has been fully worked out. Too many data items can overburden a study, adversely affecting the quality and the completeness of the items collected.

A key requirement is that the data are collected in the same setting, using identical questions. This reduces the opportunity for the location and the manner of collecting the data to influence the responses given. If data are being obtained by interview, the interviewer(s) would need to be trained to ask questions in the same way. The conditions of the interview should also be standardised. For example, if cases were interviewed in their homes where they are relaxed and comfortable, every effort should be made to do the same for controls.

One technique to encourage constancy in data collection is for the interviewer not to know whether the individual is a case or a control (i.e. be blinded). This removes any temptation to probe one group more deeply than the other. In some circumstances blinding may not be achievable, for example where the cases are bedridden or display features of an illness. Blinding can also be important when data are abstracted from records. For example, in the cerebral palsy study data were collected by reviewing the mothers' obstetric notes, ensuring that the researcher who abstracted the information was unaware if the child had cerebral palsy (3). This was intended to prevent bias: if the researcher knew which children had cerebral palsy there might have been a temptation to search more thoroughly for evidence of poor care. Alternatively the impartial researcher, determined not to fall into this trap, might overcompensate and search more diligently in the notes of the control group. Consistency of data collection is one of the major challenges of the case-control study.

ANALYSIS AND INTERPRETATION

The findings from case-control studies are commonly presented in what are called two-by-two tables. This is illustrated using data from a study of the causes of inflammatory bowel disease. One factor studied was the relationship between the use of oral moist snuff and the occurrence of disease (13):

	Ulcerative colitis cases	Controls	Totals
Used snuff	24	21	45
Never used snuff	58	124	182
Totals	82	145	227

This table shows that 29% (24/82) of the cases took oral moist snuff, but only 14% (21/145) of the controls did so. Thus those with ulcerative colitis were more than twice as likely to have used snuff as the controls. What we need to know is the increased risk of developing the disease associated with the use of snuff. It might be tempting to calculate the proportion of snuff users who have ulcerative colitis, but this would be a mistake. The answer that 53% (24/45) had the disease would be wrong, not just because it would imply that snuff use carried a massive risk of developing the disease. The fallacy in this approach can be seen by considering what would happen if there were twice as many controls as in the present study. This would increase the number of snuff-using controls from 21 to 42 (assuming the additional controls were similar to the existing ones). Now the proportion of snuff users with the disease would be 36% (24/(24+42)).

Instead of carrying out the erroneous calculation, we can use what is called an odds ratio. This gives the increased risk of developing the disease among snuff users compared to non-users. It is given by comparing the ratio of snuff users in cases and controls (24/21=1.14) to the equivalent ratio for non-users (58/124=0.47). The odds ratio is obtained by dividing the first ratio by the second (1.14/0.47)=2.4. This is simply interpreted to mean that ulcerative colitis is just over twice as likely to be experienced by users of oral moist snuff than by non-snuff-using controls. Thus, an odds ratio of 1.5 would mean that those exposed to the suspect agent were 50% more likely to develop the disease; an odds ratio of 0.5 would mean the exposed were 50% less likely to develop the disease.

The odds ratio in case-control studies is analogous to the relative risk which was calculated for cohort studies. Although these two measures are technically different, they are interpreted in the same way. The calculation of the odds ratio can be most easily explained by substituting the letters a, b, c and d for the relevant numbers. The two-by-two table then becomes:

	Ulcerative colitis cases	Controls
Used snuff	a	b
Never used snuff	c	d

and the odds ratio (OR) is given by:

OR = $a.d/b.c$

Often in case-control studies the effect of other factors needs to be taken into account. Thus in the ulcerative colitis study, cigarette smoking could be important because it was known to be protective against ulcerative colitis. Snuff users might smoke less because they could obtain nicotine without smoking, and thus be less protected against the disease. This type of effect is known as confounding, where an apparent association between two factors (ulcerative colitis and snuff) is actually due to the effects of a third (smoking). It can be taken account of by using sophisticated statistical methods which are described in the books listed at the end of this chapter. These were used in the ulcerative colitis study and the effect of snuff persisted after adjusting for smoking.

POTENTIAL PITFALLS

The findings from any type of study should be treated with some caution, but this is especially true of case-control studies. They are particularly susceptible to bias. For example, early reports that reserpine (an antihypertensive drug) could cause breast cancer led to the suggestion that treatment might need to be withdrawn in some patients. Further studies failed to confirm this relationship, leading a reviewer to conclude that the *'weak statistical association between reserpine use and subsequent breast cancer . . . is very unlikely to be one of cause and effect'* (14). More recently a controversy arose over the practice of giving vitamin K to prevent haemhorrhagic disease of the newborn. A study found that the risk of the infants developing childhood cancer was more than doubled (15). Findings from subsequent studies led an editorial in the *British Medical Journal* to conclude: *'there are considerable doubts about whether the association is causal'* (16).

The principal sources of bias in research studies (selection bias, measurement bias and confounding) are reviewed in detail in Chapter 15. But it is worth exploring here why case-control studies can be so strongly affected by them. The first reason is that case-control studies are carried out retrospectively: recent cases and controls are identified and then information is sought about events which happened some time previously. Systematic differences in their recall of past events can lead to spurious differences between cases and controls. For example, women whose babies have cerebral palsy are likely to have reviewed in some detail the course of their pregnancy and the circumstances surrounding the birth. They are thus much more likely to remember and report all sorts of events than the controls who will not have examined their pregnancy in such detail. The more distant the events on which information is being sought, the greater the chance for lapse of memory and misremembering. Data on historical events can be unreliable.

A second source of difficulty is the selection of the control group. It can be very difficult to find appropriate controls. The idea is to find controls who are as similar to the cases as possible, except that they do not have the disease or other defining characteristic of cases. Thus they should come from the same kinds of backgrounds, have similar lifestyles, and have had broadly similar medical care. The problem is that if controls are selected in a slightly different way to cases, misleading differences between them may be observed. Inappropriate control groups are a major problem for case-control studies, and great care and some skill is required to ensure this does not happen.

COMMENTS AND FURTHER READING

The case-control study can be a powerful method for research. However, it is one of the more difficult methods to use, because of the potential for minor deficiencies in study design to lead to substantial bias. This is most amply demonstrated in the title of a review paper: '*A collection of 56 topics with contradictory results in case-control research*' (17). Sources of bias in case-control studies have been reviewed by Sackett (18) and by Kopec and Esdaile (19). When the case-control is clearly the best method, the beginning researcher would be well advised to seek help from a researcher with experience of conducting this type of study. Possible candidates for help are epidemiologists and medical statisticians.

For those who wish to use this method, an excellent article on the design, conduct and analysis of case-control studies was by Mantel and Haenszel (20). Good introductory chapters to this method are also found in Lilienfeld and Lilienfeld (21), Alderson (22), and Friedman (23). More advanced texts are by Schlesselman (10), Breslow and Day (24), Rothman (25) and Kleinbaum and colleagues (26).

REFERENCES

1. Jackson, R, Scragg, R and Beaglehole, R. Alcohol consumption and risk of coronary heart disease. *British Medical Journal* 1991; **303**: 211–16.
2. Jackson, R and Beaglehole, R. The relationship between alcohol and

coronary heart disease: is there a protective effect? *Current Opinion in Lipidology* 1993; **4**: 21–6.

3. Gaffney, G, Sellers, S, Flavell, V, Squier, M and Johnson, A. Case-control study of intrapartum care, cerebral palsy, and perinatal death. *British Medical Journal* 1994; **308**: 743–50.

4. Orbell, S, Crombie, I, Robertson, A, Johnston, G and Kenicer, M. Assessing the effectiveness of a screening campaign: who is missed by eighty percent cervical screening coverage? *Journal of the Royal Society of Medicine* 1995; **88**: 389–94.

5. Arnow, PM, Bland, LA, Garcia-Houchins, S, Fridkin, S and Fellner, SK. An outbreak of fatal fluoride intoxication in a long-term hemodialysis unit. *Annals of Internal Medicine* 1994; **121**(5): 339–44.

6. Ekwo, EE, Gosselink, CA, Woolson, R and Moawad, A. Risks for premature rupture of amniotic membranes. *International Journal of Epidemiology* 1993; **22**(3): 495–503.

7. Stewart-Brown, S, Peters, TJ, Golding, J and Bijur, P. Case definition in childhood accident studies: a vital factor in determining results. *International Journal of Epidemiology* 1986; **15**(3): 352–9.

8. Darwish, MJ and Armenian, HK. A case-control study of rheumatoid arthritis in Lebanon. *International Journal of Epidemiology* 1987; **16**(3): 420–3.

9. Glass, RI, Craven, RB, Bregman, DJ, *et al.* Injuries from the Wichita Falls tornado: implications for prevention. *Science* 1980; **207**: 734–8.

10. Schlesselman, JJ. *Case-Control Studies: Design, Conduct, Analysis.* New York: Oxford University Press, 1982.

11. Schlesselman, JJ. Sample size requirements in cohort and case-control studies of disease. *American Journal of Epidemiology* 1974; **99**(6): 381–4.

12. Lemeshow, S, Hosmer, DW Jr, Klar, J and Lwanga, SK. *Adequacy of Sample Size in Health Studies.* Chichester: John Wiley & Sons, 1990.

13. Persson, P-G, Hellers, G and Ahlbom, A. Use of oral moist snuff and inflammatory bowel disease. *International Journal of Epidemiology* 1993; **22**(6): 1101–3.

14. Labarthe, DR. Methodologic variation in case-control studies of reserpine and breast cancer. *Journal of Chronic Diseases* 1979; **32**: 95–104.

15. Golding, J, Greenwood, R, Birmingham, K and Mott, M. Childhood cancer, intramuscular vitamin K, and pethidine given during labour. *British Medical Journal* 1992; **305**: 341–6.

16. Draper, G and McNinch, A. Vitamin K for neonates: the controversy. *British Medical Journal* 1994; **308**: 867–8.

17. Mayes, LC, Horwitz, RI and Feinstein, AR. A collection of 56 topics with contradictory results in case-control research. *International Journal of Epidemiology* 1988; **17**(3): 680–5.

18. Sackett, DL. Bias in analytic research. *Journal of Chronic Diseases* 1979; **32**: 51–63.

19. Kopec, JA and Esdaile, JM. Bias in case-control studies. A review. *Journal of Epidemiology and Community Health* 1990; **44**: 179–86.

20. Mantel, N and Haenszel, W. Statistical aspects of the analysis of data from retrospective studies of disease. *Journal of the National Cancer Institute* 1959; **22**(4): 719–48.

21. Lilienfeld, AM and Lilienfeld, DE. *Foundations of Epidemiology* 2nd edn. New York: Oxford University Press, 1980.

22. Alderson, M. *An Introduction to Epidemiology* 2nd edn. London: Macmillan Press, 1983.
23. Friedman, GD. *Primer of Epidemiology* 3rd edn. New York: McGraw-Hill, 1987.
24. Breslow, NE and Day, NE. *Statistical Methods in Cancer Research. Volume 1: The Analysis of Case-Control Studies.* Lyon: International Agency for Research on Cancer, 1980.
25. Rothman, KJ. *Modern Epidemiology.* Boston: Little, Brown, 1986.
26. Kleinbaum, DG, Kupper, LL and Morgenstern, H. *Epidemiologic Research. Principles and Quantitative Methods.* New York: Van Nostrand Reinhold, 1982.

Chapter 10

OTHER METHODS OF RESEARCH

Chapters 6 to 9 outline the features of the principal epidemiological methods which can be used in health services research. But there are other techniques and approaches which can be used to great advantage. This chapter reviews these methods, giving an indication of the circumstances when they are useful and an outline of their main characteristics. It does not describe in depth how to use these methods, but directs readers to more detailed texts.

QUALITATIVE METHODS

Discovering that there are deficiencies in care is often much easier than finding out why these deficiencies occur. For example, it is very easy to discover that some patients fail to keep their appointments at outpatient clinics, but uncovering the reasons for this can be much more taxing. Conventional survey methods using questionnaires might miss some of the factors involved. Because the questions would be predefined, a questionnaire would not allow individuals to explain their own thoughts and assessments. Participants would not have the opportunity to explain how they weighed each factor to arrive at their decision. This is why in-depth interviews were conducted in a study which investigated the reasons that parents failed to keep an appointment at a paediatric clinic (1). It found that: *'parents balanced the benefits of attending against the costs . . . their perception of the severity of the symptoms and of their child's prognosis was crucial in this.'* This study is an example of qualitative research.

Characteristics and Use

Qualitative research deals with descriptive data. One of its main objectives is *'to understand human behaviour from the subject's own frame of reference'* (2). The individual's perspective of a topic can be a very important one. For example, the study of people who care for a dementing elderly relative is an important area of current research. The issues it might address are: *'how carers develop a sense of their own caring role, whether they think of their relative as "demented", whether dementia represents in carers' eyes a kind of social death, and what strategies carers use to cope with their dementing relative'* (3). Investigating these would require the special techniques of qualitative research.

Qualitative research is truly exploratory. A basic tenet is that the researcher does not know what will be found, but needs to observe and interpret with care. The data collected in this type of research are the descriptions that individuals give of events, and the explanations they provide for what happened. This method focuses on individual perceptions and how these are described, *'the actor's definition of the situation'* (4). The research may also try to look behind the words being used to decipher what the person really means, what their motives or beliefs really are. It recognises that the way people behave is determined by many factors, including what they think is expected of them, how they interpret the behaviour of other people, and how they feel about what is happening.

The information gained from qualitative work may be sufficient in itself. For example, a study of women's explanations of their illnesses was able to draw valid conclusions after interviews with 23 women (5). It found that illness explanations were: *'dynamic entities that fluctuate through time in ways that allow them to be meaningfully incorporated into the mesh of ongoing life circumstances'.* In other circumstances the qualitative study may be a preliminary to a more quantitative study. This second approach was taken in an investigation of the reasons why some women did not attend for cervical screening (6). To determine the range of attitudes to screening, some 40 women were asked for their views. From these a checklist of options was prepared, on which data was systematically collected in a much larger study. It is better to determine the range of options from careful exploratory work. If researchers construct checklists by themselves, there is a danger that they may impose their own views on their subjects.

Qualitative research seeks to understand events in the context in which they happen. This can mean that the researcher is integrated into the health care setting, and must endeavour not to influence events while investigating them. The research has to be approached with an open mind: preconceptions could distort the interpretation of what is going on. This research can be carried out in a variety of ways:

- direct observation
- interview
- focus group

Direct Observation

Data can be collected by an external observer, referred to as a non-participant observer. This was the approach adopted in a study of the care of the dying, where a researcher observed doctors and nurses as they went about their duties (7). Or the data can be collected by a participant observer, who can be a member of staff undertaking usual duties while observing the processes of care. A variant on the participant observer approach is to use specially trained individuals to act as patients. This method has been used successfully (8, 9), although it is limited to conditions in which it is sufficient for patients to report appropriate symptoms; it would be of little use for conditions which should also have physical signs.

Interview

Interviews in qualitative research are usually wide ranging, probing issues in detail. They seldom involve asking a set of predetermined questions, as would be the case in surveys. Instead, they encourage subjects to express their views at length. The interviews are often tape recorded so that they can be transcribed for subsequent analysis. One useful technique is the critical incident study, in which respondents are asked to comment on real events rather than giving generalisations. This can reveal more about beliefs and attitudes and behaviour. It was used to explore the reasons why general practitioners issued certain prescriptions and what they felt about their actions (10). Patient expectation was found to be an important influence on prescribing, and failure to live up to the GP's own expectations was an important cause of discomfort.

Focus Groups

Focus groups provide another approach to qualitative research. A group of about six to ten individuals is brought together 'under the guidance of a facilitator to discuss a particular subject of common interest in a free and open manner' (11). The facilitator tries to stimulate discussion, and keep it from straying off the topic. The group size is deliberately kept small, so that its members do not feel intimidated but can express opinions freely. The technique can be used to explore opinions, ideas and issues, or to generate hypotheses. It has been relatively little used in health services research.

Comment and Further Reading

Qualitative research provides an extensive, and rapidly evolving, set of theories and methods. It is ideally suited to investigate the many subtle features of individual behaviour which affect the delivery and experience of health care. In this type of research there is less concern with obtaining representative samples of patients than is the case with surveys (see Chapter 6). This is because the research is seeking to uncover beliefs and opinions and the reasons that these views are held. It is interested in why people behave as they do rather than in estimating the proportion of individuals who hold a particular view. There are two recent books which describe the methods of qualitative research (12, 13).

Qualitative methods are particularly helpful in the early stages of a project when trying to clarify what are likely to be the important issues to be investigated. They might appear relatively straightforward, involving an open-minded observation of the delivery of care and careful interview of the staff or patients involved. However, uncovering the many subtle factors which influence human behaviour can be a very difficult task. If they are the method of choice for a research study, then it would be better to collaborate with professional sociologists, anthropologists or psychologists who have the necessary skills and experience.

ADMINISTRATIVE AND ROUTINELY COLLECTED DATA

Some research questions can be answered using data which are collected routinely. A pioneering use of routinely collected mortality data was by the nineteenth-century physician John Snow (14). He investigated cholera outbreaks occurring between 1848 and 1854. By careful analysis of the data he was able to show that drinking water taken from the River Thames, at places where it was polluted with human sewage, was able to transmit the disease.

Range of Uses

Routinely collected data provide information on the use of health care resources, and on the frequency of the different diseases. They allow the researcher to explore the way resource use and disease frequency vary from one region to another and how they change over time. They can help set the context for a project, by showing how important a disease is in terms of mortality, morbidity and resource use.

Routine data are used at a national level to decide how health care resources are to be allocated to regional health authorities. This is done using a formula which takes into account the age structure and the death rate of the local population (15). The rationale for this is that some age groups, the very young and the elderly, make disproportionate use of services so that allowance needs to be made for regions with relatively greater numbers at the extremes of age. Death rates are used as a proxy for the amount of illness in an area, which in turn should affect the need for health care.

Routine data can also help identify problems. One study showed that hysterectomy is almost three times more common in the United States than in England and Wales (16). The finding of substantial variation in the usage of health care resources has been made a number of times, within as well as between countries. It seems that differences between regions in the way health care is delivered are the rule rather than the exception. Finding the reasons for these differences is one of the major challenges for health services research.

Data on cause of death have been used to explore the impact of health care services (17, 18). The research has focused on conditions which are thought to be amenable to medical intervention. The amount of health service input is compared with the resulting mortality in different regions, to test whether additional resources lead to better outcomes. The data do provide some support for this idea, although this method of research has been challenged (19).

Types of Data

There are many sources of routinely collected data and these can be conveniently described in three categories. These are:

- mortality
- morbidity
- civil

Mortality

Annual reports on mortality are published by the Office of Population Censuses and Surveys (OPCS) in England and Wales, and by the

Registrar General in Scotland. The reports are based on death certificates from which a code for the cause of death is derived. Deaths are coded using the International Classification of Disease (ICD) (20), which also provides guidance on how to assign cause of death. The data are published separately by cause of death, age, sex, and area of residence. The World Health Organization collates mortality data from countries throughout the world, and publishes annual tables of death rates.

Morbidity

Hospital Episode Statistics are published by the Department of Health. They give details of all inpatient stays in NHS hospitals. An episode is a period of care under a consultant, so that when a patient is transferred between specialties a new episode is generated. Each patient is assigned a diagnostic code based on the ICD, and the data are published by diagnosis, age, sex, and area of residence. There are separate tables on surgical operations, and on bed usage. Data on the frequency of the various cancers, and on congenital malformations and infectious diseases, are published by OPCS.

Civil

The decennial census, undertaken by OPCS, provides the basis for population figures in the United Kingdom. Details are published of the number of people subdivided by age, sex and area of residence. Figures are also available on the number of births, marriages and divorces, subdivided where appropriate. Annual estimates of these figures are published for the intercensal years. These estimates take account of migration, births and deaths. Although the accuracy of these annual estimates will fall with increasing time from the census, in practice any discrepancies will be of little consequence.

Comment and Further Reading

Much of the routine data is primarily collected for administrative purposes and its accuracy has been regularly questioned. The concerns include the completeness of registration and the accuracy of coding. In particular, the allocation of diagnosis can be difficult, so that estimates of disease frequency from mortality and cancer incidence data should be treated with some caution.

Research using routine data more often raises interesting questions than answers them. For example, a recent study showed that the frequency of hip replacements was inversely related to the prevalence of hip pain: the higher the frequency of pain, the less likely patients were to be admitted to hospital for treatment (21). Clearly further research would be needed to understand why this paradoxical situation had occurred.

Valuable advice on the analysis and interpretation of routine data is given in many books on epidemiology, including those by Mausner and Kramer (22), Lilienfeld and Lilienfeld (23), and Alderson (24). A comprehensive review of information sources on all aspects of health, illness and health care services is given in a compendium (25). Further details on the data provided by OPCS and the Department of Health are best obtained by contacting the organisations themselves. Their addresses are:

OPCS Central Enquiries Unit
Room 502
St Catherine's House
11 Kingsway
London WC2B 6JP
Tel: 0171 396 2828

Department of Health
Skipton House
80 London Road
London SE1 6LW
Tel: 0171 972 2000

OPERATIONS RESEARCH

Operations research (OR) is not a method of investigating surgical technique. It is a specialist discipline providing a range of techniques which can be used to help plan the organisation and delivery of health care. Operations research came to prominence during the Second World War, as an aid to the design of military operations. One early use was to optimise the search for U-boats, and to determine the size of convoy which would minimise shipping losses (26). Operations research deals with complex problems where there are many possible courses of action and where there may be considerable uncertainty and risk associated with each action.

Range of Uses

Operations research has been used to study many different aspects of health care, including:

- the resource implications of cervical cytology screening (27)
- the best way of allocating blood from a regional blood transfusion service to the hospitals within its area (28)
- the likely spread of the AIDS epidemic (29)
- the flow of patients onto and out of waiting lists (30)
- the diagnosis of deep vein thrombosis (31)
- the storage and retrieval of medical records (32)
- the optimal screening policy for detecting immunity to hepatitis A (33)

These examples illustrate how operations research seeks understanding of the ways in which health care is organised and delivered. The insights provided may be used to predict future need for health care, facilitate planning, or to increase the efficiency of service delivery.

Principal Characteristics

Operations research embraces a wide range of methods, suited to the diversity of problems which it tackles. This diversity makes it difficult to provide a list of principal characteristics. Although there are common themes to these methods, the emphasis given to these varies with the application. It is easier to review the features of this method by considering two examples in more detail.

Modelling Services for Renal Disease

Patients with chronic renal failure can be managed in a variety of ways: hospital dialysis; home dialysis; ambulatory peritoneal dialysis; kidney transplant; or even no treatment. Each of these treatments makes different uses of resources, and has differing benefits for the patients. In addition, patients may move between these treatment modalities when, for example, donor kidneys become available, or when kidney grafts are rejected. It is not easy to decide how best to use health care resources to meet current need. Planning for future needs is even more difficult because innovations may change the ways patients are managed. For example, the introduction of new drugs can change the survival of patients: cyclosporin A (an immunosuppressant) increased the survival of kidney transplant patients, reducing the demand for dialysis. There could also be initiatives to increase the supply of donor kidneys, again changing the demand for resources.

The OR approach to this problem is to develop a model representing all the things that can happen to patients (34). A number of assumptions are made about how many patients are likely to enter the system, and how many will receive each of the treatments. Using computer simulation it is possible to explore what might happen in the future. The set of assumptions can be varied, for example by increasing the supply of donor kidneys, to determine the effects this would have. The model allows 'what if' questions to be asked. It can be made more realistic by recognising that new patients (like buses) do not arrive evenly spaced, but come in bunches. It can also include the different ways in which patients respond to therapy, and the differing lengths of time that each will spend on each treatment.

Deciding on Management of Suspected Deep Venous Thrombosis

A second example of the techniques of operations research deals with the management of suspected deep venous thrombosis (DVT). Many patients who present with a red, swollen, painful leg will have a deep venous thrombosis (DVT). These patients are at risk of having part of the clot break off and travel to the lungs where it may cause a pulmonary embolism. Treatment with anticoagulant therapy will reduce the risk of this, but at a price: roughly 1% of patients will suffer a stroke because of treatment. Should treatment be given? This question can be answered by working out what would happen if patients were not treated. Suppose that 40% of patients have a DVT, and that about 20% of patients with untreated DVT will suffer a pulmonary embolism. This means that about 8% of all patients will have a pulmonary embolism (20% of 40%). On balance it would seem better to treat all patients, since this would lead to many fewer suffering a serious event.

This type of calculation can be carried out using the decision tree shown in Figure 10.1. The figure shows the various events which could occur after the decision has been taken to treat or not to treat. The figure also contains the probability of these events. The probability of each possible outcome is worked out by multiplying together the probabilities along each part of the tree leading to that outcome.

In practice, the management of DVT is much more complex. Treatment does not prevent all DVT, but reduces the frequency by about one-third. There are also two types of diagnostic test which can be used to help

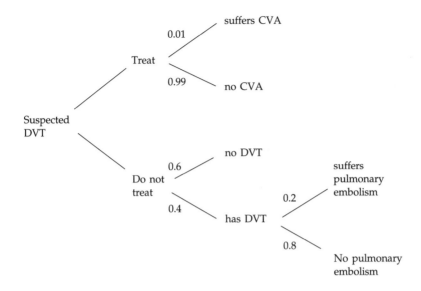

Figure 10.1 Decision tree for suspected deep venous thrombosis. Modified and simplified from Venta and Venta (31)

target treatment at patients with DVT. One is very good, but it is invasive and about 3% of patients who are examined will have a DVT induced by the test. The other test is non-invasive and carries no risk. But this test is more likely to fail to detect some clots and falsely to label patients who are clot-free as having clots. Again, this problem is approached by laying out the decision tree, assigning probabilities to the various options and calculating the probabilities of the possible outcomes. When this was carried out the surprising result was that *'the decision to treat all patients with symptomatic legs is better than doing any single test'* (31).

Common Features

The methods of OR have common features. They all try to construct a model of the part of health care being investigated. The model may simply specify the components of that part of health care and describe how they interact. Or the relationship between the components may be specified mathematically. Many models incorporate uncertainty: they allow for the play of chance (under strictly defined conditions).

Comment

Operations research provides a powerful set of tools for understanding and predicting the behaviour of complex systems. Those who use the techniques often have training in mathematics, statistics and computing. A health service researcher who felt their research question might be amenable to modelling would do well to contact a professional in this field. Many university courses on operations research involve a component of project work, thus it might be possible to involve an OR student in the research. At the least this would indicate the feasability and value of modelling the problem under study.

REFERENCES

1. Andrews, R, Morgan, JD, Addy, DP and McNeish, AS. Understanding non-attendance in outpatient paediatric clinics. *Archives of Diseases in Childhood* 1990; **65**: 192–5.
2. Shmerling, A, Schattner, P and Piterman, L. Qualitative research in medical practice. *Medical Journal of Australia* 1993; **158**: 619–22.
3. Gilleard, C. Research methods in the study of carers of dementing elderly people: a workshop report. *Health Bulletin* (Edinburgh) 1991; **49**(6): 349–51.
4. Cunningham-Burley, S. Personal communication.
5. Hunt, LM, Jordan, B and Irwin, S. Views of what's wrong: diagnosis and patients' concepts of illness. *Society of Scientific Medicine* 1989; **28**(9): 945–56.
6. Orbell, S, Crombie, I, Robertson, A, Johnston, G and Kenicer, M. Assessing the effectiveness of a screening campaign: who is missed by eighty percent cervical screening coverage? *Journal of the Royal Society of Medicine* 1995; **88**: 389–94.
7. Mills, M, Davies, HTO and Macrae, WA. Care of dying patients in hospital. *British Medical Journal* 1994; **309**: 583–6.
8. Rethans, J-J, Drop, R, Sturmans, F and van der Vleuten, C. A method for introducing standardized (simulated) patients into general practice consultations. *British Journal of General Practice* 1991; **41**: 94–6.
9. McClure, CL, Gall, EP, Meredith, KE, Gooden, MA and Boyer, JT. Assessing clinical judgment with standardized patients. *Journal of Family Practitioners* 1985; **20**(5): 457–64.
10. Bradley, CP. Uncomfortable prescribing decisions: a critical incident study. *British Medical Journal* 1992; **304**: 294–6.
11. Schattner, P, Shmerling, A and Murphy, B. Focus groups: a useful research method in general practice. *Medical Journal of Australia* 1993; **158**: 622–5.
12. Denzin, NK and Lincoln, YS, eds. *Handbook of Qualitative Research*. London: Sage, 1994.
13. Ong, BN. *The Practice of Health Services Research*. London: Chapman & Hall, 1993.
14. Hill, AB. Snow—an appreciation. *Proceedings of the Royal Society of Medicine* 1955; **48**: 1008–12.
15. Judge, K and Mays, N. Allocating resources for health and social care in England. *British Medical Journal* 1994; **308**: 1363–6.

16. McPherson, K and Bunker, J. Health information as a guide to the organization and delivery of services. In: Holland, WW, Detels, R and Knox, G, eds. *Oxford Textbook of Public Health. Volume 2: Methods of Public Health* 2nd edn. Oxford: Oxford University Press, 1991: 67–79.

17. Charlton, JRH, Hartley, RM, Silver, R and Holland, WW. Geographical variation in mortality from conditions amenable to medical intervention in England and Wales. *Lancet* 1983; **i**: 691–6.

18. Charlton, JRH and Velez, R. Some international comparisons of mortality amenable to medical intervention. *British Medical Journal* 1986; **292**: 295–301.

19. Mackenbach, JP, Bouvier-Colle, MH and Jougla, E. "Avoidable" mortality and health services: a review of aggregate data studies. *Journal of Epidemiology and Community Health* 1990; **44**: 106–11.

20. World Health Organization. *Manual of the International Statistical Classification of Diseases, Injuries, and Causes of Death* 9th revision edn. Geneva: World Health Organization, 1978.

21. Payne, JN, Coy, J, Patterson, S and Milner, PC. Is use of hospital services a proxy for morbidity? A small area comparison of the prevalence of arthritis, depression, dyspepsia, obesity, and respiratory disease with inpatient admission rates for these disorders in England. *Journal of Epidemiology and Community Health* 1994; **48**: 74–8.

22. Mausner, JS and Kramer, S. *Mausner & Bahn. Epidemiology: An Introductory Text* 2nd edn. Philadelphia: W B Saunders Company, 1985.

23. Lilienfeld, AM and Lilienfeld, DE. *Foundations of Epidemiology* 2nd edn. New York: Oxford University Press, 1980.

24. Alderson, M. *An Introduction to Epidemiology* 2nd edn. London: Macmillan Press, 1983.

25. Morton, LT and Godbolt, S. *Information Sources in the Medical Sciences* 4th edn. London: Bowker-Saur, 1992.

26. Cretin, S. Operational and system studies. In: Holland, WW, Detels, R and Knox, G, eds. *Oxford Textbook of Public Health. Volume 2: Methods of Public Health* 2nd edn. Oxford: Oxford University Press, 1991: 345–62.

27. Boyd, A, Davies, LA and Bagust, A. Modelling the implications for hospital services of cervical cytology screening: a case history. *Journal of the Operational Research Society* 1989; **40**(6): 529–37.

28. Sapountzis, C. Allocating blood to hospitals. *Journal of the Operational Research Society* 1989; **40**(5): 443–9.

29. Roberts, C and Dangerfield, B. Modelling the epidemiological consequences of HIV infection and AIDS: a contribution from operational research. *Journal of the Operational Research Society* 1990; **41**(4): 273–89.

30. Worthington, D. Hospital waiting list management models. *Journal of the Operational Research Society* 1991; **42**(10): 833–43.

31. Venta, ER and Venta, LA. The diagnosis of deep-vein thrombosis: an application of decision analysis. *Journal of the Operational Research Society* 1987; **38**(7): 615–24.

32. Liu, C-M, Wang, K-M and Guh, Y-Y. A Markov chain model for medical record analysis. *Journal of the Operational Research Society* 1991; **42**(5): 357–64.

33. Farrington, CP. Optimal screening policies for Hepatitis A. *Journal of the Operational Research Society* 1989; **40**(4): 355–9.

34. Davies, H and Davies, R. A simulation model for planning services for renal patients in Europe. *Journal of the Operational Research Society* 1987; **38**(8): 693–700.

Chapter 11

SELECTING THE METHOD

Chapters 5 to 10 have reviewed the variety of research methods which are available for health services research. This variety brings with it the problem of selecting the most appropriate method for a given research question. In some instances more than one method could be used successfully to answer a particular question. But often one will achieve the desired aim more quickly and with much less effort than the others. The methods have different strengths, but also have their own weaknesses and limitations. Thus the method chosen will not just be the one which will be the easiest to use, but which will also provide valid conclusions. This chapter provides guidance on how to select the best method for a given research question. It does so by reviewing the primary uses of each method together with the main limitations.

STAGES IN SELECTING A METHOD

Identifying the best method for research involves reviewing and critically appraising the potential methods to determine the most suitable. There are a number of steps in identifying possible methods:

- refine the question
- review the literature
- review the methods in turn

Refine the Question

The key to the selection of the best research method is to make sure that the research question has been fully worked out. The process of doing this is described in Chapter 3, but in brief it involves asking: What do I really want to find out? Often when this has been clarified the research method is readily apparent. But even if the method appears obvious, it is worth reflecting on other possibilities. Making the wrong choice at an early stage is a surefire method of storing up trouble for the future.

Review the Literature

One way to identify likely methods is to review the literature for instances when others have tried to answer similar research questions. If a method has already been used successfully, then it has a good chance of working in a further study. Published reports sometimes comment on the nature and degree of difficulty which was encountered in the study. They may also point out the limitations which the study design imposes on the interpretation of the findings. Less commonly, reports may suggest alternative ways of answering the same question. However, some authors are reluctant to say that an alternative method would be preferred because it raises the awkward question: Why didn't you use the better method to start with? Thus even when a method has previously been used, it is worth considering whether another might be more suitable.

Review the Methods in Turn

Research questions can be grouped according to the type of method which could be used. Table 11.1 does this for some of the types of questions which are commonly asked in health services research. This table can help narrow the search, matching particular research questions to those listed in the table. The table also shows that for many questions more than one method could be used. In practice, deciding which method to use involves taking each method in turn and asking: Could this be used to answer the question?

Could it be a Survey?

Surveys are ideal for describing what is going on now. They can be used to describe the types of patients being seen at clinic, or the characteristics of nurses who undertake research. Surveys can also be used to give an estimate of how many people have some condition: for example the number of undiagnosed asthmatics in the community.

Surveys are one of the most commonly used methods of health services research, but there is a danger that they may be inappropriately used. When ideas for research first present they are often in the form: '*I want to find out more about this topic.*' Phrased in this way it might seem that a survey would be the natural choice of research method. In many instances surveys will be a suitable method (see Chapter 6). But there will be other times when one of the other research designs is more

Table 11.1 Potential methods for some typical research questions

Research question	Method
What kinds of:	
● patients attend this clinic?	
● persons care for disabled relatives?	survey
● nurses undertake research?	
How many:	
● persons have undiagnosed asthma?	
● doctors use this treatment?	survey
● patients are satisfied with their treatment?	
What happens:	
● to patients admitted to A&E?	
● to doctors after qualification?	cohort
● after patients are discharged?	
What are the long-term:	
● survival rates?	
● complications of this disease?	cohort
● health needs of patients?	
What happens following:	
● stroke rehabilitation?	
● postgraduate education?	cohort/clinical trial
● day case surgery?	
Is this treatment more effective than that?	clinical trial
Why do some patients:	
● fail to comply with treatment?	case-control study/
● develop complications?	cohort
● have extended inpatient stays?	
What do patients believe:	
● about the causes of their illness?	qualitative methods/
● about the treatments they have received?	survey/case-control study
How do we predict:	
● future demand for health care?	operations research
● the effect of changes in health service delivery?	
How do we determine:	
● the factors which influence waiting lists?	operations research
● the best way to organise service delivery?	

appropriate. Do not rush into a survey simply because it looks as if this method will provide useful data.

Surveys are particularly deficient in answering research questions which involve an element of time. This can be most easily seen by taking a somewhat extreme example. Suppose a researcher wanted to find out how long patients have to wait for a kidney transplant. One approach would be to survey those receiving a transplant and ask about the length of wait. However, the answer would be misleading because it would omit all those who had died prior to receiving a transplant. The selective loss of fatal events would also distort estimates of the types of patients receiving a transplant. Older patients would be more likely to die from other causes and would be relatively under-represented in the sample studied. Surveys describe the state of events at a point in time, but in looking at events over time they are bedevilled by selective loss.

Could it be a Cohort Study?

Cohort studies are best suited to finding out what happens over time. Consider again the investigation of patients waiting for a kidney transplant. In addition to finding out how long patients wait for a donor organ, the researcher might well be interested in asking: Do some types of patients wait longer than others? Do those who wait longer have a poorer outcome? These questions involve following patients to see what happens to them. The element of time in these questions means that they are best answered by cohort studies (Chapter 7).

Cohort studies do not only identify current patients and follow them into the future. They can identify patients from past records and follow them until the present (or to some convenient date). This was the approach adopted in a study to determine whether patients admitted to hospital with a diagnosis of schizophrenia are at an increased risk of developing cancer (1). Patients were identified from stored hospital records, and followed through time for up to 37 years. The study found that the risk of suicide was increased tenfold, but there was no increase in the risk of cancer. The extended period of follow-up was needed because cancers can take many years to develop. Thus the only feasible way to conduct the study was to identify patients admitted to hospital many years previously.

An important limitation of cohort studies is in assessing the effectiveness of therapies. At first sight it might seem that the natural way to decide if a treatment is effective would be to give it to a group of patients and monitor how well they fare. But using cohort studies to answer questions of effectiveness is problematic. The reasons for this were explored in some depth in Chapter 8, but in brief they turn on the difficulties of interpreting the results. To decide whether the treatment has worked, patients need to be compared with a group receiving some other therapy. The two patient groups need to be similar prior to treatment so that fair comparisons can be made. This seldom occurs in practice. In most circumstances the clinical trial is the preferred method of assessing effectiveness.

Could it be a Clinical Trial?

Research questions which should be answered using a controlled clinical trial (Chapter 8) are relatively easy to identify. Clinical trials are used to compare the effectiveness of treatments, or of different approaches to management, or even the effectiveness of staff training programmes. The research question will often contain the term 'effective', or can be rephrased to include this term. Consider the following examples of research questions: Does GP education improve outcome for patients with chronic asthma? Does geriatric rehabilitative care reduce the length of stay of patients with hip fracture? Can a linkworker increase the uptake of breast cancer screening? Does counselling the whole family help childhood obesity? Does biofeedback reduce the number of episodes of stress incontinence?

All these questions could be recast into the form: Is the proposed intervention effective? They have all been addressed using clinical trials (2–6). A common feature of these studies is that they all assessed effectiveness by comparing the proposed intervention with an alternative. What is being asked is not Does it work?, but instead Does it work better? A fair comparison can only be made when patients are recruited then randomly allocated to receive one or other treatment. Random allocation is one of the hallmarks of the clinical trial, which makes it the method of choice for questions of effectiveness.

There are many circumstances in which a clinical trial might be desirable, but could not be used because it would be unethical. For example, there is suggestive evidence that breast feeding may augment the mental development of children (7). The best way to resolve this issue would be to allocate newborn babies randomly to receive either breast or formula milk. But it would be unethical to deprive some babies of the known advantages of breast milk (such as the passive immunity acquired from the mother). Thus the research is conducted using cohort studies which are recognised to suffer from bias and confounding. In consequence the issue is still in doubt.

Could it be a Case-control Study?

A question which is commonly asked in health services research is: Why are these patients different? When the intention is simply to obtain a broadbrush description of the patients, then a survey may be sufficient. This would be the case if all that was wanted was a general picture of factors such as their age, gender, disease duration and severity. But when the interest lies in determining why they differ from other patients, then a control is needed (so that comparisons can be made). This is the basis of a case-control study. For example, a group of researchers wanted to know whether medical exposure to anaesthetic gases could be associated with the development of Alzheimer's disease (8). The finding that Alzheimer's patients had had an average of 188 minutes of general anaesthetic could not be interpreted in isolation. It leaves unanswered whether this is more, or indeed less, than might be expected. By incorporating a control group in their study the researchers were able to show that the exposure was no higher than that experienced by other patients of the same age who did not have this disease. In general the case-control design (Chapter 9) provides a sensitive method of asking the question *'why?'* It is a useful method of investigating events which occur after a long interval, such as the development of Alzheimer's disease. It is also well suited to the investigation of rare events.

The limitations of case-control studies arise partly from the difficulty of identifying appropriate controls (see Chapter 9). Doubts about the suitability of the controls bedevil the interpretation of study results. There can also be concerns over the validity and reliability of the data, especially when information is being collected about events which took place some time ago. In the Alzheimer's disease study the information is likely to be recorded in casenotes and would be reliable. Clearly, it could not be obtained by asking the patients. Doubts about the controls and the quality of the data combine to weaken the usefulness of case-control studies.

Is a Qualitative Technique Required?

Qualitative methods (see Chapter 10) are best suited to in-depth exploration of the beliefs, attitudes and motivations of patients and health care professionals. They can tease out the complex web of factors which influence behaviour. In some circumstances a qualitative study is conducted as a prelude to a survey, cohort or case-control study. It is used to identify the key issues which are then investigated in a larger quantitative study.

Could Routine Data Help?

A key element of many research studies is the issue of the scale of the problem being investigated: How big a problem is it? Is it worth investigating? This may be answered by estimates of the frequency of the disease or the numbers of patients who die from it. Alternatively, the importance of the problem may be reflected in the extent of the usage of health care resources. Questions of this nature can be answered using routinely collected administrative data (see Chapter 10)

Does the Study Involve Service Planning?

A common concern in health care is how best to organise the delivery of care to maximise the number of patients treated. When research poses questions of the form: What will happen if we introduce a new service? or What is the best way of organising this service? the method of choice is likely to involve some of the techniques of operations research (see Chapter 10).

SELECTION IN PRACTICE

Reviewing the possible methods in turn may still leave a choice between two apparently suitable methods. The decision between these often involves balancing theoretical and practical considerations. The relative importance of these factors will vary between studies.

An Example of Selecting

Consider a study to investigate factors which might influence the risk of having a stillborn baby. This could be approached using a case-control or a cohort study. The case-control study would compare women who had had a stillbirth against those whose babies were liveborn. Cases could be identified from hospital records. Controls could be healthy infants matched by sex and date of birth and obtained from the discharge records from the same hospitals. The problem facing the case-control study lies in obtaining data on potential risk factors during pregnancy. Information from the casenotes could be used, but that would restrict the data set to those variables which were routinely recorded. Questioning women who had stillborn babies would raise ethical concerns, but these could be overcome if a counselling service were provided. A more intractable problem is one of bias. Women who had lost a baby might tend to review their pregnancies in detail, searching for explanations of their loss. They are much more likely to recall and report events during pregnancy which women with healthy babies might overlook. This could produce associations between events and stillbirths which were artefactual.

A cohort study on this topic would not be affected by the problem of recall bias. Pregnant women could be identified at the time of their first attendance at antenatal clinic. Details of their pregnancy would be recorded at interviews on each subsequent visit until full term. The information could be recorded without bias because no one would know which women would have a stillbirth. But the cohort study faces the problems of size and cost. Stillbirth is a rare event, and many hundreds of women would need to be followed up to have a sufficiently large study. Almost all the women followed up would have healthy babies, resulting in the collection of considerable amounts of unnecessary data. This problem would be compounded by the amount of interview data which would be collected at each of the antenatal visits.

Which method should be chosen? The case-control study would be much cheaper to carry out. Unbiased data could be obtained by reviewing the medical records of a comparatively small number of cases and controls. But this would restrict the factors which could be investigated. It would exclude behavioural factors such as the diet, exercise, stress and even medical events such as colds and flu which might not be routinely recorded in casenotes. The cohort study could collect this additional information, but at a price. This would be worth paying if the researchers believe that these latter factors were likely to be the important ones. Thus the choice of method depends crucially on what the study is trying to find out, as well as the practical problems likely to be encountered during the study.

Pulling it Together

The stillbirths example showed how different methods can be reviewed in turn to identify the factors on which each is weak. The types of questions being asked are:

- How difficult will it be?
- What will it cost?
- How likely is bias to occur?

The answers to these questions will vary greatly with the specific study to be conducted, but some general comments can be made. Case series are usually easy to conduct, whereas case-control studies and clinical trials are often difficult. These difficulties reflect the complexities of the study designs. Surveys and cohort studies vary in their degree of difficulty: they can be very difficult in some instances but much easier in others. Drawing up an outline study design, indicating what has to be done and when, will quickly indicate how complex a study is likely to be.

The practical difficulty of a study will depend on how easily the participants can be contacted and recruited, how easily the required measurements can be made and the data collected, and the length of time required to complete the study. An assessment of these practical issues can be made by inspecting the detailed study design and asking of each item: How do I do this? Tasks which appear straightforward often turn out to be much more difficult than expected. Thus if an activity appears difficult at first sight, in practice it may well be impossible.

The likely costs of studies are largely determined by their degree of difficulty, with case series and clinical trials being at opposite ends of the spectrum. But two other factors come into play when considering case-control studies and cohort studies: the size of the study and the time it will take to complete. Other things being equal, cohort studies require to be much larger than case-control studies. They can also take considerably longer if patients need to be followed up for any length of time.

The likelihood of bias reflects the amount of experimental control which the researcher has. Bias is potentially greatest in case series because of the unknown selection which can influence the group being studied. It is least in clinical trials: the study group is well defined; patients are randomly allocated to active treatment or control; and there is blinded assessment of outcome. Thus valid comparisons can be made. In contrast, case-control studies are much more subject to bias because of the difficulties of obtaining an adequate control group and of gathering information retrospectively.

The practicability of a study may not be fully apparent when it is being planned. But if it seems that the method might work, try it out on a very small scale to see if it really is feasible. There is nothing like a pilot study for revealing the shortcomings of a research design.

COMMENT

The selection of a method has been presented as a linear sequence, beginning with a research question, passing through theoretical considerations and finishing with practical ones. In reality, the researcher will constantly move between these stages, seeking potential methods as the research question is being refined, and searching out possible flaws in these methods. These considerations will frequently help refine the research question, leading to one for which there is a valid and feasible method. However when the method has been finally selected, it is worth asking one final time: Can we do it? Will it work? Are there serious flaws? Research studies take time and effort. They should only be undertaken when there is a good chance that they will work.

REFERENCES

1. Saku, M, Tokudome, S, Ikeda, M, *et al.* Mortality in psychiatric patients, with a specific focus on cancer mortality associated with schizophrenia. *International Journal of Epidemiology* 1995; **24**(2): 366–72.
2. White, PT, Pharoah, CA, Anderson, HR and Freeling, P. Randomized controlled trial of small group education on the outcome of chronic asthma in general practice. *Journal of the Royal College of General Practice* 1989; **39**: 182–6.
3. Kennie, DC, Reid, J, Richardson, IR, Kiamari, AA and Kelt, C. Effectiveness of geriatric rehabilitative care after fractures of the proximal femur in elderly women: a randomised clinical trial. *British Medical Journal* 1988; **297**: 1083–6.
4. Flodmark, C-E, Ohlsson, T, Rydén, O, Sveger, T. Prevention of progression to severe obesity in a group of obese schoolchildren treated with family therapy. *Pediatrics* 1993; **91**(5): 880–4.
5. Hoare, T, Thomas, C, Biggs, A, Booth, M, Bradley, S and Friedman, E. Can the uptake of breast screening by Asian women be increased? A randomized controlled trial of a linkworker intervention. *Journal of Public Health Medicine* 1994; **16**(2): 179–85.
6. Burns, PA, Pranikoff, K, Nochajski, TH, Hadley, EC, Levy, KJ and Ory, MG. A comparison of effectiveness of biofeedback and pelvic muscle exercise treatment of stress incontinence in older community-dwelling women. *Journal of Gerontology* 1993; **48**(4): M167–74.
7. Florey, CdV, Leech, AM and Blackhall, A. Infant feeding and motor development at 18 months of age in first born singletons. *International Journal of Epidemiology* 1995; **24** (Suppl. 1): S21–S26.
8. Bohnen, NILJ, Warner, MA, Kokmen, E, Beard, CM and Kurland, LT. Alzheimer's disease and cumulative exposure to anesthesia: a case-control study. *Journal of the American Geriatrics Society* 1994; **42**(2): 198–201.

Chapter 12

RELATED DISCIPLINES

Health services research is a broad discipline which embraces a wide range of activities, and employs a variety of methods. It is characterised by diversity, and draws heavily on the skills and expertise of other disciplines. This chapter provides an introduction to the most important of these related disciplines. It does so primarily to signal their existence and to indicate in brief the ways in which they can contribute to health services research. The intention is to illustrate their potential within health services research, rather than to provide a full or systematic coverage.

HEALTH ECONOMICS

Health economics provides a way of thinking and a set of tools to help decide whether specific health care activities are financially worthwhile. It helps to clarify how health care resources should be spent to best advantage. The intention is to ensure that the maximum increase in health gain is obtained for a given level of expenditure.

Range of Uses

The discipline of health economics is sometimes thought to have emerged relatively recently, but it dates back several centuries. One of the earliest recorded uses was in London in the seventeenth century, when plague was a major cause of mortality. It was recognised that the number of deaths could be reduced by moving people to the countryside while the epidemic raged in the city. The question was whether the cost of this would be justified by the wealth generated by the labours of those who would be saved. A somewhat crude calculation showed that: *'every pound expended would yield a return of £84'* (1).

Health economics has two cardinal features: the cost of an activity or process; and the health gain which results from it. These can be seen in a number of recently published studies which have asked the following questions:

- Is the cost of giving kidney patients hepatitis B vaccination prior to dialysis justified by the reduction in infection rates? (2)
- Does the cost of antimicrobial prophylaxis in dental practice outweigh the reduction in the cases of infective endocarditis? (3)
- Is urinary catheterisation better (in terms of costs and effects) than incontinence pads for the management of intractable urinary incontinence? (4)
- Which method of screening for Down's syndrome represents the best value for money? (5)
- Is the extra cost of an air suspension bed outweighed by the reduction in the frequency of pressure sores? (6)

These examples illustrate the two central calculations in health economics: the cost of what is done and the benefit which results. It is worth reviewing the assessment of costs and the measurement of health gains in a little detail.

Assessing Cost

The assessment of cost is the easier of the two calculations in health economics, but it still presents a formidable array of problems. The process involves several activities:

- identify the sources of cost
- assign costs
- limit the sources of cost
- consider the complexities

Identify the Sources of Cost

The sources of costs can be identified by reviewing the activities involved in supplying care. Consider the costs of repairing a fractured neck or femur using a surgical implant (7). In addition to the cost of the implant itself, allowance must be made for theatre costs, hotel costs (food, laundry, bed), medical costs (including investigations and treatments), ward costs and overheads (such as hospital records department, managerial staff, heating and lighting). The identification of all potential contributors to cost can require thorough exploration of all the services which patients may receive. For example, the hip patients may require laboratory investigations, blood transfusions, X-rays and electrocardiographs, and may be visited by physiotherapists, occupational therapists and social workers. Identifying all these costs will involve considerable work.

There is an important distinction between what are termed fixed and variable costs. Fixed costs are those which must be paid no matter how many patients are treated. These include the capital cost of buildings and equipment, and the salaries of some staff, for example those required to maintain equipment and essential services. Variable costs are those which depend on the level of activity, such as the amount of food eaten, the number of tests ordered, the number of drugs prescribed.

In some circumstances it may be relevant to include the costs incurred by the patients and their family and friends. Economics takes a wide view of costs, and considers not only out-of-pocket expenses like travel to the hospital, but also loss of wages because of absence from work.

Assign Costs

Having identified all the relevant sources of costs, a value has to be assigned to each. This is where the difficulties really begin. Consider assessing the cost of treating hip fracture patients. The cost of some items, such as the implant used or the drugs given, could be obtained from hospital purchasing records. Other types of cost, for example the overhead costs, would have to be divided up among all the patients treated, possibly in proportion to the length of each patient's stay. Apportioning costs is especially tricky for capital costs, like hospital buildings or expensive pieces of equipment. For these items the capital costs have to be weighed against the length of time for which they will be used, to calculate the portion which should be assigned to each patient.

Some of the difficulties of assigning costs can be overcome by using published estimates for the costs of items such as bed days in different types of accommodation (e.g. intensive care, acute medical, rehabilitation) or for standard costs of operations and other procedures. In practice, these average costs have to be used with some care. Costing can be a difficult business, with many hidden complexities.

Limit the Sources of Cost

The variety of possible contributors can make costing extremely difficult. This will always be the case when the total costs and consequences of a health care intervention are to be assessed. Thus research which asks questions such as: What is the total cost of this service? will be difficult to undertake. The process of costing can be greatly simplified if the research focuses on only a part of the health care given. This might involve comparing alternative ways of delivering the same service. For example, one study investigated whether peripheral parenteral nutrition was cheaper than the alternative method of using a central venous catheter (8). The costing data were restricted to the process of catheterisation: setting up the line; maintaining the line; and dealing with complications. All other health care costs could be ignored as they would be the same for both types of management. Peripheral nutrition, known to be a lower risk procedure, was shown to be a cheaper alternative as well.

Research focusing on the consequences of changing the way a service is organised can also simplify the task of costing. One group looked at the consequences of increasing the interval between follow-up appointments in a diabetic clinic (9). This would free some appointment times at which new patients could be seen, increasing the total number of patients seen. There would be increased costs for clerical staff (arranging the extra appointments) and an increased use of blood and urine tests. But many other costs would be unaltered, including: the buildings and equipment; the salaries of doctors and nurses; and the travel costs of patients attending (if the total number of patient appointments is unaltered the travel costs will be unaltered, even if a larger number of patients is making the visits). The study showed that increasing the interval between appointments from seven to nine months would almost double the number of patients who could be seen, with only a 5% increase in cost.

The benefits of a focused research question were highlighted in Chapter 3. The same general approach applies in health economics: do not try to cover all costs, but refine the research question to limit the sources of cost. In doing this the types of questions being asked are: What is the aspect of health care that I am really interested in? What can I compare it with to simplify the process of costing?'

Consider the Complexities

The costs of health care activities are not fixed, but can vary depending on a number of different factors. For example, the costs of a diagnostic test usually fall as the number being performed rises: a consequence of economies of scale. Further, when a service is first introduced it will tend to be more expensive as staff have new and difficult tasks to perform. As they gain experience, they will become more efficient. A dramatic example of this was seen with heart transplantation. In one American hospital the cost of the first operation was estimated at $81 000, which fell to $48 000 by the tenth operation and to $25 000 by the fiftieth (10).

Averages costs may show, for a given service, the level of expenditure for each patient treated. But they are less useful for questions of the form: How much will it cost to treat an extra three patients a week? When buildings and equipment are already in place and trained staff are in post, the cost of treating a few extra patients will be substantially less than the average cost. The actual additional cost of treating each extra patient is termed the marginal cost. It may only involve a small increase in staff time, a few diagnostic tests and the prescription of some drugs. However, in other circumstances the increase in patients seen could have a substantial effect: it might mean an extra outpatient clinic, or the opening of a new ward to accommodate the additional patients.

A second area in which average values can be misleading is in the estimation of the costs of length of patient stay. The most expensive part of a patient's stay occurs in the first few days, when investigations and operations are being carried out. Towards the end of their stay, many patients are convalescing and will require only some nursing care and hotel facilities. It would clearly be a mistake to assume that trimming a day or two off the end of a stay would generate the level of saving indicated by the average cost for the whole episode of treatment.

There is a further problem. Reducing length of stay may transfer some of the burden of care from the hospital to the community. Thus costs will be borne by the primary care sector and by family and friends of the patient. Estimating all these costs considerably broadens the area of study.

Summing up Costs

Costing is often a complex business. The above discussion has outlined two important principles. The most appropriate costs to use are marginal costs: the actual cost which results from the proposed increase (or decrease) in activity, e.g. what it actually costs to treat a few extra patients, given that the facilities and staff are available. Secondly, economists often take a very broad view of costs: to include those accruing to primary care, to social work services, to family and friends, and even to loss of work opportunity. Because of these complexities, some care should be given to the casting of the research question to simplify the process of costing. This can involve comparing the costs of different ways of providing a service, or assessing the impact of changes to the organisation of care. The advantage of these approaches is that many sources of cost can be ignored.

Measuring Health Gain

Health care can have a wide range of intended results: for cancer patients the intention may be to prolong life, unless the illness is terminal when the intention is to reduce suffering; for hypertension, the immediate aim is to reduce blood pressure, with the longer-term aim of preventing strokes and heart attacks; for schizophrenia, therapy may be aimed at controlling symptoms. Thus a number of different health gains can be distinguished, depending on whether the intention is to reduce the:

- duration of disease
- frequency of disease recurrence
- frequency of death
- severity of symptoms
- levels of disability

Health economics can thus assess benefit in a variety of ways, which are often presented in three groups:

- clinical events
- quality of life
- monetary value

Clinical Events

The easiest method of assessing health gain is to focus solely on clinical outcome: the number of extra years of life lived as a consequence of treatment; the number of cases of disease diagnosed as a result of a new screening test; the number of cases of disability prevented. This approach is limited by the paucity of information about the effectiveness of many health care interventions. As has been noted in earlier chapters, much health care is based on convention rather than evidence. However, the current movement to evidence-based medicine may see this limitation overcome.

Quality of Life

An extension to counting clinical events is to look at the quality of the health gain. For example, a new technique might save the lives of some patients with very severe stroke. The value of the technique would depend not just on the number of extra years of life lived, but also on the level of long-term disability. If many of the patients saved by the new management plan were unable to walk, talk or feed themselves, a lower value would be placed on the new service. Quality of life reflects the World Health Organization definition of health: *'a state of complete physical, mental and social well-being and not merely the absence of disease or infirmity'* (11). Many standardised questionnaires have been developed to measure quality of life. Some are general purpose and can be used for many different patient groups, while others have been developed for particular types of disease. Many of the widely used questionnaires are described in books by Bowling (12, 13) and Wilkin and colleagues (14).

Monetary Value

Economists take the assessment of outcome one stage further: they estimate the monetary value of the health gain which results from treatment. This means that a cost has to be assigned to each of the types of health gain identified above. For an outcome such as death, one strategy is to calculate the income which the person would have earned had they lived to the normal retiring age. This is an old technique, used in the seventeenth century to investigate the value of providing lying-in beds in hospital for the birth of illegitimate children (1). The cost of thirty days' inpatient stay, then the recommended period, was estimated at thirty shillings (£1.50 in present day units). This was reckoned to be substantially less than the value of the labour that would be gained from these children when they matured. The argument was strengthened by noting that 30 shillings was much less than the price being paid for Negro children in the American plantations.

The loss of income approach has limitations. How can a monetary value be ascribed to pain, or to loss of the ability to walk or feed oneself? Economists have developed a number of approaches to overcoming these problems (15). These require individuals to place values on health and illness. One technique is to ask individuals how much they would pay not to suffer from an illness. This was applied to patients with rheumatoid arthritis, who, on average were willing to lose some 22% of their household income to be free of their disease. This approach appears to allow members of society to determine for themselves the value placed on health care services. However, the results will depend on personal circumstances. A person who has a disease, or has a close relative with the disease, will value services for that disease more highly than will those with no experience of the disease. The amount that individuals are willing to pay will also depend on the number of financial commitments they have and on personal attitudes to health and disease. Assigning a monetary value to human well-being is a complex and problematic business.

Economic Assessments

Economists have developed a number of different techniques for evaluating health care. These are:

- cost minimisation
- cost effectiveness
- cost–utility
- cost–benefit

Cost Minimisation

There is often more than one way in which a patient can be managed: hip fracture patients could have planned early discharge or conventional management; patients with kidney disease could have renal dialysis or renal transplantation; gastric ulcers could be treated by surgery or by drug therapy. Cost minimisation can be used to decide between such alternatives. It assumes that the alternative approaches are equally effective, i.e. each produces a similar amount of health gain. This assumption will seldom be met in practice, so that this method can seldom be used.

Cost Effectiveness

Cost-effectiveness analysis is a natural development of cost minimisation: it takes into account the differences in effectiveness of alternative treatments. The focus is again on differing approaches to the same end. For example, stroke patients could be managed in a general medical ward (the cheaper alternative) or in a specialist stroke unit (the more effective). The alternatives could be compared by calculating the cost in pounds sterling for each additional life saved. This technique is limited by the lack of good data on the effectiveness of the alternative approaches. In the case of stroke, there have been several studies comparing specialist units against conventional management. But for many of the instances where there is more than one form of management, comparative evidence is lacking.

Cost–utility

Health services are frequently faced with decisions like: Should these extra resources be allocated to neonatal intensive care or outpatient facilities for rheumatoid arthritis patients? These activities result in quite different health gains: the first will save lives, the second will reduce disability and suffering. They cannot easily be compared. One solution is to convert all health gains into the same units. In principle, this can be achieved by measuring the years of life gained by a particular intervention and the quality in each of those years (16).

The use of QALYs (Quality Adjusted Life Years) in determining health care priorities has been criticised (17), and economists acknowledge its deficiencies (18, 19). It depends crucially on estimates of quality of life and life expectancy, information which is often unavailable. Nonetheless, it is likely that QALYs, or some equivalent measure, will increasingly become a part of the health service in the future.

Cost–benefit

Cost–benefit analysis extends the cost–utility approach by assigning a monetary value to the benefits of health care. It does so using the types of techniques described above in the section on costing. Estimating monetary values of health gain presents problems at least as formidable as those encountered when estimating quality of life. A recent review of this technique concluded that currently *'its usefulness is limited'* (20).

Comment and Further Reading

Economic evaluation is being seen more frequently in health services research, and the trend is more likely to accelerate than abate. There will be increasing concern to obtain the greatest possible health benefit with the limited resources available for health care. Advances in medical research often lead to more expensive techniques for investigating and treating patients, and demand for treatment seems always to grow.

The practice of economic evaluation is far from straightforward. Many factors contribute to this, including the plethora of contributors to costs; the need to use marginal costs rather than average ones; the difficulties of assessing health gain; and the many dimensions of quality of life. Some journals have run series of articles on health economics (16, 20–27) and there are helpful textbooks (15, 28).

In the face of these difficulties, the researcher would need to keep studies as simple as possible, and seek advice from a professional economist whenever possible. The simpler studies involve either cost minimisation or cost effectiveness. These approaches minimise the difficulties of estimating health gain. Studies can be further simplified by selecting specific aspects of patient management, rather than trying to cost the entire episode of health care delivery. Restricting economic evaluation in this way must be done with some care, lest there be important costs or health gains beyond the focus of the study. Economic evaluation should be handled with care. There is much to commend the view that the principal contribution of health economics is the conceptual tools it supplies and the emphasis given to the need to examine costs and benefits (17).

HEALTH PSYCHOLOGY

Psychology involves the study of behaviour. The term psychology derives from the Greek word *psyche* meaning mind or self. Psychological factors are central to health care, affecting the demand for it, as well as its organisation and delivery. This statement can be made without equivocation: consider the impact of genital herpes on a teenage girl, of mastectomy on a mature woman, or the detection of the HIV virus in a healthy young man. In each there can be an immediate powerful emotional reaction, and long-term psychological distress. In short: *'emotional and other psychological reactions are an integral part of physical well-being and the process of medical care'* (29). Psychology is the discipline which provides understanding of people's experiences and their behaviour.

Range of Uses

Psychology can contribute to many aspects of health care delivery. Some examples of recent studies include the assessment of:

- the communication and counselling needs of patients with lymphoma (30)
- the factors which determine the effectiveness of self-management of diabetes (31)
- the attitudes, intentions and behaviours of blood donors (32)
- the importance of psychological factors in the occurrence of multiple allergy (33)
- the strategies patients adopt to cope with a diagnosis of cancer (34)
- the attitudes of GPs to persons with epilepsy (35)

These examples illustrate the increasing recognition of the central role of psychological factors in health and health care delivery. The issues include: why some individuals adopt unhealthy lifestyles; why patients seek medical help; why doctors manage patients in the way they do; why some patients fail to comply with therapy; how people can be encouraged to adopt health-promoting behaviours; how people cope with their illnesses. Thus psychology contributes to our understanding of people's:

- lifestyle
- care seeking
- attitudes and beliefs about illness
- response to illness
- coping strategies
- relationship with health care professionals

It can also provide understanding of the attitudes and beliefs held by health care professionals. These insights enable us to predict behaviour and also suggest how it can be modified.

The Strengths of Psychology

Psychology provides formal methods to observe behaviour, to derive explanations for the behaviour, and to test those explanations. The benefit of these formal methods is to limit the opportunities for making mistakes. An example will help illustrate how easy it is to misinterpret observations of behaviour. In the 1930s, '*it was fashionable in many hospitals to discourage parents from visiting their children*' (36). This policy was thought reasonable at the time, because it had been observed that many children became upset when their parents left. In consequence, reducing the number of visits would reduce the amount of upset. Subsequent study showed that many of the children suffered emotional disturbance on being reunited with their parents, and the effects of maternal deprivation are now more fully recognised. Current policy is to provide accommodation for a parent to stay with an ill child.

Psychology provides a wealth of evidence on the factors which affect behaviour, together with a body of theory to help interpret and predict behaviour. For example, it has been established that behaviour is influenced by feelings, emotions, attitudes, beliefs and moods. A number of models have been proposed to explain behaviour, one of which is the health belief model (37). This proposes that an individual's health-related behaviour depends on an assessment of their susceptibility to disease and the potential severity of the disease if it were contracted. A behaviour will be adopted if its benefits (reduction in susceptibility or potential severity) outweigh possible barriers (financial, physical or psychological costs). This model was used in an investigation of the reasons some women do not attend for cervical screening (38). It explored whether those who did not attend thought they were at reduced risk of the disease. It also investigated the importance of potential barriers, such as difficulties of getting to the screening clinic or the anticipated discomfort or embarrassment of the screening test. The model helped identify specific ideas to be tested, and it clarified the types of data which should be collected. In general models will often contribute to research studies in both these ways. The challenge is to identify and select the model most appropriate to the research question. This is best achieved by asking a professional psychologist.

Another strength of psychology derives from the array of techniques which have been developed to measure all aspects of behaviour. A number of standardised instruments (often in the form of questionnaires) are available to measure intelligence, stress, anxiety, and depression as well as attitudes and beliefs. For example, a study of chronic pain patients used the Beck Depression Inventory to determine the association between depression, pain intensity, and the effect which pain had on the lives of the patients (39). It found that patients with depression suffered greater pain and experienced more disruption to their lives.

Questionnaire-based instruments are relatively easy to use but, as there are many different ones available, it can be difficult to decide which is most appropriate. There are also many different dimensions of health and well-being, for each of which there are a range of instruments. A recent textbook reviewed 11 measures of psychological well-being, 10 measures of life satisfaction, and 12 measures of general health status, among many others (12). In addition, there will be many specialist instruments for use on specific patient groups. When deciding on which questionnaire to use, it would be well worth contacting a researcher experienced in the use of these instruments.

Comment

Health psychology has a great potential within health services research, but to date this has been little realised. A traditional criticism of psychology is that its findings are little more than common sense: 'all psychology is doing is stating in abstruse language some fairly obvious everyday knowledge' (40). In part this may be an example of the application of hindsight: when a new explanation is proposed which is immediately sensible there may be a tendency to think: 'Well yes of course, that is obvious.' But without careful research the obvious finding might never have been realised.

There will also be many situations in which subtle but important factors would be overlooked were it not for the contribution of psychology. An example of this is the study of users and non-users of cervical screening (38). Although factors such as anticipated embarrassment and discomfort were common among the non-users, they were also seen among the users, albeit to a lesser extent. But a major difference between users and non-users was whether the anticipated problems would act as barriers to attendance. It was found that, although the users of cervical screening anticipated these problems, this was unlikely to deter them from attending for screening. The non-users considered the same problems to be major impediments to attendance. The study thus identified the barriers which health education would need to address to improve the uptake of cervical screening.

Psychology is a distinct and well-established discipline, and this text can only provide a brief introduction to it. Whenever a research study starts asking questions of the form: Why do they do that? What makes them behave in that way? the researcher would be well advised to seek advice from a professional psychologist, or perhaps a medical sociologist.

MEDICAL SOCIOLOGY

Medical sociology is concerned with the social context of health, disease, illness and health care delivery. Social factors play a crucial part in illness and its management. Even the apparently clinical issue of whether a person has a disease can be socially determined. For example, alcoholism used to be regarded as a form of socially deviant behaviour, but is now seen as a disease which should be treated. In contrast, pregnancy outside marriage was regarded in the early part of the twentieth century as a sign of mental illness, and many unfortunate women were consigned to asylums because they had a baby when unmarried. The clinical characteristics of alcoholism and pregnancy have not altered; it is the way society, and particularly health professionals, view them which has changed.

The contribution which sociology has to offer is sometimes dismissed because '*it only tells you what was obvious to start with*'. One of the most elegant refutations of this is contained in the work of Lazarsfeld (cited by David Tuckett) (41). Six supposed findings are presented, each with a comment to explain why it is correct. One example was that men from a rural background, because they are more accustomed to hardship, adapt more easily to army life than soldiers from a city background. All the statements appeared to fit into the category '*obvious to start with*', but each was the direct opposite of what was actually found. Perhaps more surprisingly, when the true results were stated, with the accompanying rationale, they again appeared obvious. Social behaviour is much more complex and subtle than it appears, and our intuitive interpretations of it can be woefully wrong.

Range of Uses

Medical sociology can investigate the way health care is organised and the interactions between the professional groups who deliver it. It asks questions like: What are the characteristics of the groups involved? What are the social and professional mores of each group? What form do the relationships between professional groups take? What implications do these findings have for the delivery of health care? Two crucial concepts underlying the approach of medical sociology are status and role. The professional status of doctors, and the differences in status between house officers and consultants, are easily recognised. Each status position has rights and obligations associated with it, and it is expected that individuals with a given status will act in particular ways to fulfil certain roles. Consultants can direct the activities of more junior doctors, but are expected to teach them and to take ultimate responsibility for patient care. Difficulties can arise when a professional group views its rights and obligations in a different way to another group. A dramatic instance of this conflict of perspectives is the confrontation between a doctor requesting an expensive drug to treat a dying patient, and the administrator with an overspent drug budget trying to balance this request with a dozen others. Often the conflict can be more subtle, and can occur within a professional group, or even within an individual. Each person plays many roles, whether as doctor, wife, mother, colleague, teacher or friend, and conflicts often occur between them: Do I stay longer with a bereaved relative (professional carer), and thus arrive home after my children have gone to bed (parent)?

Another important area of medical sociology is the lay perspective on health, the views of the sick and the healthy in the general population. The questions posed might be: What kind of health care do people want? How do they go about getting it? How do patients view their illnesses? How does illness affect patients' lives? One of the early findings in medical sociology was of the *cultural and social structural impediments to the effective use of the available technology of medicine*' (42). These went a long way to explaining why some patients do not consult a doctor, and why others do not attend follow-up appointments or comply with recommended treatment. Central to the study of these issues is the view that the attitudes and behaviours of individuals cannot be understood without considering the social group to which the individual belongs. Humans are social animals and much of their behaviour is governed by the values and expectations of the groups to which they belong. If most of your friends are smokers then it can be difficult to remain a non-smoker. Similarly, if there is a shared view that a treatment is ineffective or carries unacceptable side effects, then patients may not seek medical attention. People behave according to their social context; transferred to a different setting, they may act quite differently. This can be seen by considering your own behaviour in contrasting settings. How much different would it be in church compared to a football match, or in your parents' home compared to your own home? In health care delivery the contrasts may be less obvious but the same principles apply.

The sociological approach also emphasises that disease does not just make a patient unwell: it can also affect their ability to take part in normal social activities, and can have consequences for their family and friends. A natural extension of this broader approach to the impact of disease is to ask which groups in society become ill, and why the prevalence of disease is higher in some groups than others. The concern here is not with the biological determinants of disease (viruses and bacteria, pollutants in the environment, etc.), but with the social factors (for example, unemployment, social class, ethnicity, stress, social support). The questions being asked are: How do social factors mediate disease? What are the health care needs of the various social groups, and to what extent are these being met? What changes are needed in the organisation of health care to redress social inequalities in health? These are all valid research areas for medical sociology.

Strengths of Sociology

Sociology provides a theoretical basis for understanding the way society is structured, the factors influencing the attitudes and beliefs of individuals, and how these interact to influence individual behaviour. Faced with a medical problem, the sociologist will naturally ask a quite different, but nonetheless important, series of questions than the clinician. For example when faced with the current issue of injecting drug use and the risk of HIV infection, the clinician might be interested in the burden that AIDS will present to the health service, the extent of spread of HIV infection into the wider community, and the opportunities for preventing diseases like pneumonia to which AIDS patients are particularly susceptible. In contrast the medical sociologist might ask: What has been the response of the health professions to the problem? Why have needle exchange schemes been more fully employed in some areas than others? What do drug users know of the risks of HIV? Why do some drug users share needles? How do the views of peer groups influence views on HIV risk? What influence does HIV risk have on the sexual behaviour of drug users?

The discipline of sociology provides a range of methodologies for studying these phenomena: direct observation, informal interviewing, semi-structured and structured interviewing. It has garnered a wealth of experience for the conduct of these types of study. These skills are not just needed for the study of emerging epidemics like HIV and AIDS, but are frequently called for in health services research. For example, the development of guidelines for the management of asthma, recently produced by a number of professional bodies (43), is clearly a clinical concern. However, when the interest is to disseminate these guidelines to the health professionals, asthma support groups, and to the patients themselves, medical sociology can help.

Comment

There is clearly considerable overlap between medical sociology and health psychology. Both deal with the way individuals behave, and they can use similar methods in their study of this. But there is a difference of emphasis. Sociology places more weight on the interaction between individuals and the impact of social conditions and social factors on health and the use of health services. The distinction can be seen by considering the factors which influence whether those with a medical problem seek professional help. Psychologists would be interested in the interpretation the patient places on their symptoms and on the likely benefit the patient anticipates from the visit, the other courses of action which the patient could take (self-medication, alternative medicine), and on the personal costs of seeing the doctor (e.g. inconvenience, embarrassment, fear of confirmation of serious disease). Sociologists would also be interested in health and illness in the context of daily life: whether the views of family and friends affect the decision, and how social interpretation of disease and the doctor–patient consultation is viewed.

The sociological approach can be employed to great advantage in health services research. But it can be difficult for the non-sociologist to use its methods or take advantage of its theories. In general, if the research begins to involve asking: Why do that group of patients/health professionals do that? How can we change the way things are done? then it might be worthwhile contacting a medical sociologist.

HEALTH PROMOTION

Health promotion, in a variety of guises, has been undertaken within the health service for many years. One of the most longstanding examples is antenatal care. Pregnant women are given advice on many topics: diet, exercise, smoking, alcohol, and dental hygiene, with the aim of enhancing their own health and that of their babies. The emphasis is on empowering them to do so, by giving both knowledge and encouragement.

Antenatal care illustrates that health promotion involves much more than dealing with disease and ill-health; it is concerned with the patient's well-being. This broad concept includes living a fulfilling life, having control over one's life, and being *able to choose what one wants to do or be, and of being able to develop one's talents'* (44).

The Range of Health Promotion

Health promotion comprises three overlapping spheres of activity (44):

- education
- prevention
- protection

These spheres can be illustrated in the context of antenatal care. Health education is more than just giving information about health and illness. It means providing learning opportunities to enable individuals to choose healthy lifestyles: avoiding health risk and adopting health-enhancing behaviours. In antenatal care women are not just given leaflets about good diet, but have nutritional advice interwoven into talks about pregnancy, foetal development and childbirth. Prevention comprises a set of actions to prevent disease or other unwanted outcome; whether this is preventing pre-eclampsia in pregnancy, or supplying contraceptives to prevent further pregnancies. Protection is the least self-evident of the three spheres, but can be broadly described as the sum of government policies and actions which promote health. In antenatal care examples of protection include the provision of maternity leave, and government policy to provide free dental care during pregnancy and for some time after the baby is born.

The Challenge for Health Promotion

In health services research, health promotion will primarily involve education and prevention aimed at patients. (Opportunities for protection are most probably limited to leaders of the profession who may be able to influence government policy. Equally, initiatives aimed at the general population will usually be undertaken by full-time health promotion workers.) The scope for health promotion will depend on the clinical setting, but the common question to ask is: What types of patient behaviours could be encouraged to improve health and well-being? Patient compliance with therapy is one ready target, especially in chronic diseases like asthma and diabetes where it is often poor.

The challenge in all of this is: How do you get people to do what's good for them? (45). Although a full exploration of the answers to this question is beyond the scope of this book, some helpful advice is:

* do not blame victims
* work with patients
* find the barriers
* offer solutions
* agree goals
* keep it simple

When patients do not comply with therapy, or eat foods which may harm them (for example eating spicy foods if they have an ulcer), there is a tendency to think *'Well, it's their own fault.'* This is unhelpful. Instead, the reasons why patients behave in this way need to be understood, and measures taken to work with the patient to achieve more healthful behaviour. Possibly the patient didn't understand the advice given previously. It is too easy to give unhelpful advice like *'eat the right food'*, without explaining which of the items that the patient eats could be harmful and what the consequences of eating them might be. It might also be that social pressures, from family and friends, make it difficult to comply even if the patient is willing. Deciding which of these factors contributes to behaviour can be difficult. Once again, we are in the realms of psychology and sociology. Recognising this means that appropriate advice can be sought. The challenge is not just to identify the important factors influencing patient behaviour, but to develop successful strategies to influence these.

Evaluation

Whenever health promotion is undertaken, the critical question is: Does it work? It can be easy to design educational packages which look as though they should work, but this is no guarantee that they will. The ideal method of evaluating any package is the randomised controlled trial in which patients would be randomly allocated to be given or not given the health promotion (see Chapter 8 for details of this method). This method is only likely to be of use for evaluating new strategies: for existing ones there are likely to be ethical and practical difficulties in withholding advice and information from half the patients. An alternative approach is to assess particular aspects of the programme asking patients whether they: Like it? Read it? Understand it? Remember it? Act on it? This can help identify where the strategy breaks down and how it might be improved.

Comment

Health promotion is a discipline whose importance is being increasingly recognised. There are a number of helpful books on the design and evaluation of health promotion strategies, including those by Downie and colleagues (44), by Ewles and Simnett (46), and by Naidoo and Wills (47). Within the NHS there is a growing body of expertise in health promotion. Each health authority has a health promotion unit whose staff can provide advice and support to those planning their own health promotion exercises.

REFERENCES

1. Fein, R. On measuring economic benefits of health programmes. In: McLachlan, G and McKeown, T, ed. *Medical History and Medical Care.* London: Oxford University Press, 1971: 181–220.
2. Oddone, EZ, Cowper, PA, Hamilton, JD and Feussner, JR. A cost-effectiveness analysis of hepatitis B vaccine in predialysis patients. *Health Service Research* 1993; **28**(1): 97–121.
3. Gould, IM and Buckingham, JK. Cost effectiveness of prophylaxis in dental practice to prevent infective endocarditis. *British Heart Journal* 1993; **70**: 79–83.
4. McMurdo, MET, Davey, PG, Elder, M-A, Miller, RM, Old, DC and Malek, M. A cost-effectiveness study of the management of intractable urinary incontinence by urinary catheterisation or incontinence pads. *Journal of Epidemiology and Community Health* 1992; **46**: 222–6.
5. Shackley, P, McGuire, A, Boyd, PA, *et al.* An economic appraisal of

alternative pre-natal screening programmes for Down's syndrome. *Journal of Public Health Medicine* 1993; **15**(2): 175–84.

6. Inman, KJ, Sibbald, WJ, Rutledge, FS and Clark, BJ. Clinical utility and cost-effectiveness of an air suspension bed in the prevention of pressure ulcers. *Journal of the American Medical Association* 1993; **269**(9): 1139–43.

7. Hollingworth, W, Todd, C, Parker, M, Roberts, JA and Williams, R. Cost analysis of early discharge after hip fracture. *British Medical Journal* 1993; **307**: 903–6.

8. May, J, Sedman, P, Mitchell, C and MacFie, J. Peripheral and central parenteral nutrition: a cost-comparison analysis. *Health Trends* 1993; **25**(4): 129–32.

9. Jones, RB and Hedley, AJ. Adjusting follow-up intervals in a diabetic clinic: implications for costs and quality of care. *Journal of the Royal College of Physicians London* 1986; **20**(1): 36–9.

10. Woods, JR, Saywell, RM Jr, Nyhuis, AW, Jay, SJ, Lohrman, RG and Halbrook, HG. The learning curve and the cost of heart transplantation. *Health Service Research* 1992; **27**(2): 219–38.

11. World Health Organization Interim Commission. Constitution of the World Health Organization. *Chronicle of the World Health Organization* 1947; **1**(1–2): 29.

12. Bowling, A. *Measuring Health: A Review of Quality of Life Measurement Scales.* Buckingham: Open University Press, 1991.

13. Bowling, A. *Measuring Disease: A Review of Disease-Specific Quality of Life Measurement Scales.* Buckingham: Open University Press, 1995.

14. Wilkin, D, Hallam, L and Doggett, M. *Measures of Need and Outcome for Primary Health Care.* Oxford: Oxford University Press, 1992.

15. Drummond, MF, Stoddart, GL and Torrance, GW. *Methods for the Economic Evaluation of Health Care Programmes.* Oxford: Oxford University Press, 1987.

16. Robinson, R. Cost-utility analysis. *British Medical Journal* 1993; **307**: 859–62.

17. Klein, R. The role of health economics [editorial]. *British Medical Journal* 1989; **299**: 275–6.

18. Gerard, K and Mooney, G. QALY league tables: handle with care. *Health Economics* 1993; **2**: 59–64.

19. Carr-Hill, RA and Morris, J. Current practice in obtaining the "Q" in QALYs: a cautionary note. *British Medical Journal* 1991; **303**: 699–701.

20. Robinson, R. Cost–benefit analysis. *British Medical Journal* 1993; **307**: 924–6.

21. Robinson, R. What does it mean? *British Medical Journal* 1993; **307**: 670–3.

22. Robinson, R. Costs and cost-minimisation analysis. *British Medical Journal* 1993; **307**: 726–8.

23. Robinson, R. Cost-effectiveness analysis. *British Medical Journal* 1993; **307**: 793–5.

24. Robinson, R. The policy context. *British Medical Journal* 1993; **307**: 994–6.

25. Lowson, K. Health economics for clinician managers. *Clinician in Management* 1993; **2**(2): 8–10.

26. Lowson, K. Health economics for clinician managers. *Clinician in Management* 1993; **2**(3): 9–12.

27. Lowson, K. Health economics for clinician managers. *Clinician in Management* 1993; **2**(4): 8–10.

28. Mooney, GH, Russell, EM and Weir, RD. *Choices for Health Care. A Practical Introduction to the Economics of Health Provision* 2nd edn. Basingstoke: Macmillan Press Ltd, 1986.

29. Friedman, H and DiMatteo, M. *Health Psychology*. Englewood Cliffs: Prentice-Hall, 1989: 3.
30. Fallowfield, L. Communication and counselling needs of patients with lymphoma. *British Journal of Hospital Medicine* 1994; **52**(2/3): 70–3.
31. Goodall, TA and Halford, WK. Self-management of diabetes mellitus: a critical review. *Health Psychology* 1991; **10**(1): 1–8.
32. Cacioppo, JT and Gardner, WL. What underlies medical donor attitudes and behavior? [editorial]. *Health Psychology* 1993; **12**(4): 269–71.
33. Howard, LM and Wessely, S. The psychology of multiple allergy [editorial]. *British Medical Journal* 1993; **307**: 747–8.
34. Dunkel-Schetter, C, Feinstein, LG, Taylor, SE and Falke, RL. Patterns of coping with cancer. *Health Psychology* 1992; **11**(2): 79–87.
35. Frith, JF, Harris, MF and Beran, RG. Management and attitudes of epilepsy by a group of Sydney general practitioners. *Epilepsia* 1994; **35**(6): 1244–7.
36. Mackay, CK. *Introduction to Psychology*. Basingstoke: Macmillan Education, 1973: 10.
37. Mullen, PD, Hersey, JC and Iverson, DC. Health behavior models compared. *Social Science and Medicine* 1987; **24**(11): 973–81.
38. Orbell, S, Crombie, I, Robertson, A, Johnston, G and Kenicer, M. Assessing the effectiveness of a screening campaign: who is missed by eighty percent cervical screening coverage? *Journal of the Royal Society of Medicine* 1995; **88**: 389–94.
39. Haythornthwaite, JA, Sieber, WJ and Kerns, RD. Depression and the chronic pain experience. *Pain* 1991; **46**: 177–84.
40. Burns, RB. *Essential Psychology: For Students and Professionals in the Health and Social Services* 2nd edn. Lancaster: Kluwer Academic Publishers, 1991: 2.
41. Tuckett, D. Sociology as a science. In: Tuckett, D, ed. *An Introduction to Medical Sociology*. London: Tavistock Publications Ltd, 1976: 43–73.
42. Freeman, HE and Levine, S. The present status of medical sociology. In: Freeman, HE and Levine, S, eds. *Handbook of Medical Sociology* 4th edn. Englewood Cliffs: Prentice-Hall, 1989: 1–13.
43. Anonymous. Guidelines on the management of asthma. *Thorax* 1993; **48** (2 Supplement): S1–24.
44. Downie, RS, Fyfe, C and Tannahill, A. *Health Promotion: Models and Values*. Oxford: Oxford University Press, 1990.
45. Sarner, M. Marketing health to Canadians. *Health Education* 1984; (Fall): 2–9.
46. Ewles, L and Simnett, I. *Promoting Health: A Practical Guide* 2nd edn. London: Scutari Press, 1992.
47. Naidoo, J and Wills, J. *Health Promotion: Foundations for Practice*. London: Baillière Tindall, 1994.

Chapter 13

ISSUES IN DATA COLLECTION

Data collection is one essential process which is common to all methods of research. It sometimes appears a simple process: for example it might only involve compiling a questionnaire which is posted to a selected set of patients. In practice, the data collection needs to be planned with some care. Beginning prematurely can lead to essential items being omitted and to errors in some of the items collected. Data collection involves three major activities: deciding which data items to collect; choosing how best to measure these items; and selecting the best method of collecting them. This chapter reviews these activities from the perspective of the researcher: beginning with a research question and working step by step to produce a defined set of data items and a clearly described method of obtaining them.

IDENTIFY THE DATA TO COLLECT

Deciding which data items to collect is a crucial but difficult task. The answer to the question how many items should be collected is: *'as many as necessary and as few as possible'* (1). To ensure that all the essential items and few inessential ones are collected, it is helpful to follow a systematic process of listing, reviewing, rejecting and re-reviewing the items to be collected. This process involves a number of stages:

- specify the study aims
- list the important factors
- review subject description
- review the literature
- prune with vigour
- check the data will meet the aims

Specify the Study Aims

Data collection begins with a clear statement of the study aims. The logic of this is: *'to be sure of arriving at your destination, first make sure you know exactly where that is'*. When the study aims are clearly specified, they should point to a list of the key items to be collected. For example, a study was carried out to determine the natural course of whooping cough. It was prompted by concern that the publicity given to this disease had created the view that it was *'always severe, debilitating and dangerous'* (2). This presumption could increase the difficulty of diagnosing mild or moderate disease, reducing the opportunity for treatment and the prevention of spread. The aim of the study then was to determine the severity and debility associated with the disease. Thus the key items to be collected were measures of severity and debility. In general, if the key items are not immediately obvious then the research question and study aims should be clarified using the approaches described in Chapter 3.

List the Important Factors

Having identified the key items, consideration can be given to the types of factors which might be related to them. The idea is to identify those factors which could influence the key items, or help explain how the results came to be as they are. In the case of the whooping cough study, attention focused on why patients differed in severity of disease, and what kinds of distress were suffered. It found that non-immunised patients suffered more severe disease, and that the most distress was experienced by the parents of the severely ill patients. The general approach to identifying these factors is to review each key item in turn, asking questions such as: What can influence this? Who else might be affected? Who will be affected most?

Review Subject Description

Certain items of data are collected because they provide a description of the study subjects, even though they may not be directly relevant to the study aims. For example, when studying patients it would be natural to collect items like age, sex, address, social class, source of referral, and duration of disease. These would enable the researcher to say what the patients are like, so that others could decide whether the findings were likely to be applicable to their patients. It is difficult to provide general rules about which items are needed for a description of study subjects. This will depend largely on the context of the study, on whether factors such as area of residence or social circumstances are relevant. One way of identifying these descriptive variables, as well as other important items for inclusion in the study, is to review the literature.

Review the Literature

Previous studies will usually have gone through the same process of searching for important items, and will have addressed the problem of how best these items can be measured. Often they will have identified important items which others might have overlooked. The checking of published reports is not an alternative to the review of data items: researchers must satisfy themselves that they have reviewed the topic thoroughly. But a research study would be severely criticised for omitting an item which had previously been shown to be important.

Prune with Vigour

The first stage of data collection involves creating a list of items for possible inclusion in the study. The next involves deciding what to discard. Although the distinction between essential and unnecessary data items depends primarily on the research question being asked, there are two categories of item which can frequently be omitted without loss:

- irrelevant clinical detail
- the 'might be interesting' items

One way to view the way the mind stores information is as a series of barrels with bungs in the bottom. For each barrel a certain key word will knock out the bung, so that all its contents are released. Those who have marked student examination papers will have seen this phenomenon at work: one word from an examination question will produce a cascade of information, most of it irrelevant. Clinical terms in a research question often have a similar effect: they stimulate the collection of all the items which are clinically relevant to the key term, whether or not they are needed for the research. It can be quite difficult to resist the temptation to do this. The breadth of knowledge of health care professionals is such that items which are clinically related to the research question will often put themselves forward during the stage of study design. Clinical detail in a study should always be critically reviewed to determine which items are really necessary to answer the question.

When reviewing potential data items for a research study, many items will frequently present themselves in the guise of: Wouldn't it be interesting to measure this as well? Indeed, it might prove interesting, or alternatively it could be a complete waste of time. There are always many interesting items which could be collected, but attempting to collect them all can overburden a study. The cost of collecting the item needs to be weighed against the chances of it adding to the major findings of the study. It is sometimes argued that since the study is being done anyway, it won't cost any more to collect a few extra items. This is only true when the number of extra items is indeed small, and their collection in no way interferes with the main purpose of the study. But the quality of data can deteriorate as the effort of obtaining them increases, so add extra items with care. Any item collected in the uncertain hope that it might be interesting is a strong candidate for exclusion.

Collaborative studies are particularly susceptible to collecting unnecessary items. It is often difficult to convince colleagues that their pet item should not be collected. But the argument is not whether the item is potentially interesting, but whether it is essential for the current study. Health services research faces enough difficulties without adding to them by collecting non-essential data.

Check the Data Will Meet the Aims

When a list of data items has been compiled and pruned, it should then be reviewed against the stated aims of the study. The intention is to see how the data items map onto the individual aims. This should show whether sufficient data have been collected to meet each of the aims. Deciding which data to collect can involve substantial time and effort, and it is relatively easy to overlook or discard some items which are essential to one of the aims. Thus before finalising the list of data items, a final check should be carried out to ask: Do we have all the data items needed to meet each of the study aims?

DECIDE HOW TO MEASURE

Many data items are easily measured. Height, weight, age and blood pressure can all be easily obtained. But many other items present challenges for measurement. Tackling these can involve several different activities:

- convert the general to the specific
- consider indirect measures
- review the quality of the data items

Convert the General to the Specific

Often the way an item is first couched presents difficulties for data collection. For example, disease severity is a term which is easy to state but less easy to define. What is wanted is a list of the items from which disease severity can be gauged. In the whooping cough study these were the occurrence of vomiting, whooping, apnoea, and complications and the number of paroxysms (2). Using this checklist of symptoms the study found that most cases of whooping cough were relatively mild.

Health services research will often encounter the need to convert general factors into specific items which can be easily measured. For example, patient satisfaction may appear a simple idea, but gaining useful information on it can be difficult. Research has shown that there are many different dimensions of satisfaction, including difficulties of access, the patient's assessment of the humaneness, informativeness and competence of the medical staff, the continuity of care and the outcome of the therapy (3). Separate questions would need to be addressed to each of these, as patients may well be satisfied in some areas but less satisfied in others. The same levels of complexity may also be encountered when measuring other facets of patients' experience such as quality of life, levels of disability, and ability to carry out activities of daily living. These experiences are conventionally measured by questionnaires consisting of a number of separate questions. The answers to these questions can be combined to produce an aggregate score. Many of the available quality of life questionnaires have been reviewed in two recent books (4, 5).

Social class, and its counterpart deprivation, are two factors which are strongly related to ill-health and death. Social class can be measured by an individual's occupation, by assigning types of jobs to the different social classes (6). It can also be measured by educational attainment, or current income or by combinations of occupation, education and income. A comprehensive review of these differing measures of social class is given by Liberatos and colleagues (7).

Consider Indirect Measures

Indirect measures are commonly encountered in medicine: body temperature is taken as a measure of fever; blood glucose as a measure of diabetic control. They are used as proxies for the underlying disease process which cannot be measured directly. In research, indirect measures are used when it is difficult to measure directly the item of interest. For example, slow intestinal transit has been associated with diseases like large bowel cancer, gallstones and diverticular disease. But the best way to measure transit time, using radio-opaque markers, is a lengthy procedure and exposes subjects to radiation. An imaginative alternative is the Bristol Stool Form Scale, which uses the stool consistency (ranging from 'hard like nuts' to 'fluffy pieces with ragged edges') as an indirect measure of transit time. Research has shown that untrained observers can provide accurate estimates of transit times using this scale (8).

Indirect measures can be used in a variety of circumstances. For example, collecting information on the control of symptoms in asthmatic patients can present problems. One solution might be to provide patients with a diary in which they could record episodes of wheezing and breathlessness, but there would remain concerns about the completeness of recording. A simpler alternative would be to monitor the use of aerosol inhalers on the basis that a high consumption of β-agonist is an indicator of poor control. Similarly the consumption of morphine, a drug widely used for the control of cancer pain, has been used as a measure of the adequacy of palliative care. Many countries were found to use very little morphine, suggesting that *'3.5 million cancer patients suffer needlessly'* (9).

Biochemical measurements can also be used as indirect measures. For example, sulphide concentrations of mouth air have been shown to be a reliable and sensitive measure of halitosis (10). The amount of urea in the breath has been widely used to detect the presence of *Helicobacter pylori*, taking advantage of the bacterium's propensity for producing large amounts of a powerful urease enzyme (11). Cotinine is a metabolite of nicotine and can thus be used to estimate the extent to which individuals have been exposed to cigarette smoke. It can be measured on a saliva sample and is a very sensitive measure of smoking exposure. One study in schoolchildren found that saliva cotinine increased progressively with the number of persons in the household who smoked (12).

Many of the factors of interest in health services research may not be amenable to direct measurement. But some imagination (and, more often, a review of others' efforts) may provide an alternative measure which can be obtained more simply.

Review the Quality of the Data Items

Part of the process of deciding how to measure the selected items should involve assessing the quality of the data being collected. There are many different aspects of quality, and attention needs to be given to:

- requirements for accuracy
- reliability
- validity
- need for sensitivity
- cheapness and ease of use

Requirements for accuracy

Before investigating whether a data item is accurate, it is helpful to decide the level of accuracy required. In research it is never possible for data to be completely error free. There will always be errors in the measuring. Instead of complete accuracy, what is needed is for the data to be good enough for the purposes of the study. Consider a study which involves finding patients' weights. To be accurate patients would have to be completely undressed, but this will present practical and personal difficulties. Some compromise will be needed where patients are allowed to retain sufficient clothes to preserve modesty, but not to wear heavy jackets or jerseys which would substantially distort the weight. The issue then is whether small inaccuracies, caused for example by wearing a few light garments, can be tolerated. This will depend on the uses to which the measurement is to be put. If it is to be used to allocate patients to broad weight categories (such as light, average or heavy) then errors of the order of one or two pounds would not matter. However, if the measurements were being used to record weight loss following treatment, then an error of a few pounds could be crucial.

Errors can be tolerated when they are likely to have only a very small effect on measurements, particularly when correcting the error would involve substantial effort. Thus some attempt should be made to assess the likely size of the errors, so that their impact can be determined. If errors can be easily prevented this should be done. But when it is difficult or expensive to eliminate an error this should not be attempted: instead, the magnitude of the error should be reduced to what is reasonable given the purposes of the study.

Reliability

A reliable measurement is one which when repeated gives a similar result on each occasion. There are a number of reasons for results varying from one occasion to the next. People vary from one day to the next, and some change more quickly than that. Thus physical measures such as blood pressure or peak flow respiration will differ over time. People's moods and attitudes also vary over time, and thus they are likely to give differing answers to questions.

The circumstances in which the measurements are taken can also influence the results. Blood pressure is one example of this, varying with body position, stress and exercise. It is recommended that a quiet room be used and that patients remain at rest for at least five minutes (having avoided stressful activities for an hour). The pressure should be measured on the right arm (it has a higher pressure than the left one), and that arm should be supported (13).

The person collecting the data can also contribute to the variation between measurements, the effect of observer error. Feinstein (14) has provided an extensive bibliography on observer error. Observers will differ in the information they obtain from patients, the interpretation of the results of tests, the findings made at clinical examinations, the resulting diagnoses. The more a measurement relies on judgement, the greater the scope for observer error.

When poor reliability is suspected it can be investigated by taking measurements on two occasions. This can be particularly important when making a measurement for the first time, or when using a newly developed questionnaire. The difference between the two measurements can be calculated and compared with the size of effect that the study is trying to detect. If errors are large enough to be troublesome then the conditions of measurement may need to be standardised. This would involve reviewing the factors which might influence the measurement. Standard conditions of measurement could then be defined, so that consistent data are obtained. The staff may also need explanation and training in the techniques of measurement.

The need to standardise the collection of data does not just apply to taking measurements, it is equally important for all types of data collection. Information needs to be collected systematically on all subjects in a study, be they people, casenotes, or hospital trolleys. If questions are being asked of people, they must be asked in the same way each time. If casenotes are to be reviewed, this must be carried out with the same diligence every time. The motivation is to obtain high quality information for all those selected for study.

Validity

A valid measurement is one which measures what it is supposed to measure. For example, the results from a questionnaire on alcohol consumption would have to be treated with some caution because some people may understate their true consumption. There will always be doubt about the validity of questions on sensitive personal issues like sexual activity, diet and personal hygiene.

Poor validity arises when the results obtained are consistently different to those which should have been obtained. Consider what would happen if a slightly deaf person were measuring blood pressure using a sphygmomanometer. As the cuff pressure is gradually lowered the observer identifies systolic pressure at the point at which a clear tapping sound is heard. This will occur at a lower pressure for a slightly deaf person than one with normal hearing. If diastolic pressure is taken at the point when all sounds disappear, this will occur at a higher pressure for a slightly deaf person. Thus the observer described would consistently underestimate systolic pressure, while overestimating diastolic pressure.

Sometimes data are not collected on certain aspects of health behaviour because of doubts about their validity. For example, to assess their skills in the use of condoms, volunteers were asked to place a condom on a transparent acrylic penile model (15). It was thought that certain aspects of condom skills (whether the package was opened carefully or torn roughly using teeth; whether the condom was unrolled before being placed on the model) might accurately reflect true behaviour. However, it was thought that the participant's ability to remove the condom from the model was unlikely to resemble the real-life situation.

In general, the validity of measurements should always be reviewed. They can be formally assessed in a number of ways (for a full review see references (1, 16)) but only three are considered here. These are:

- face validity
- content validity
- criterion validity

Face validity involves asking for each data item: How likely is it that we are really measuring what we want? Suppose a researcher wanted to investigate whether patients were having difficulty sleeping. It might appear that this could be investigated by asking: On average how many hours did you sleep in hospital? But this would take no account of individual need for sleep, the quality of the sleep, the number of disturbances during sleep, nor whether the patient felt rested after the sleep. Thus the examination of face validity involves an informal review of the proposed measure, asking: Does it get to the nub of the issue? Are all aspects covered? What could be missed? How could it give misleading answers?

Content validity applies when dealing with multi-item questionnaires. For example, when assessing physical function of patients with rheumatoid arthritis, patients might be asked about their ability to walk on the flat, climb stairs, dress themselves, take a bath, use the toilet, and clean their teeth. The important issue is whether all the appropriate elements have been included in the questionnaire. Other items which might be considered important for physical function include the abilities to open bottles and jars, to hang out washing, and to fill and pour from a kettle. Content validity can only be assessed after a detailed review of the topic being investigated, to check that all relevant items are being collected. The question of exactly what is wanted will depend on the purposes of the study.

Criterion validity compares the results which have been obtained against some gold standard. For example, a questionnaire designed to detect psychiatric disorders was tested against a standardised psychiatric interview (17). It was able to detect about 85% of the cases of psychiatric illness which were diagnosed clinically. Criterion validity is the most important of the measures of validity, but its use is often limited by the lack of gold standard measures to compare against.

Need for Sensitivity

There are usually different ways of measuring a data item and these can vary in sensitivity. Suppose a researcher was studying chronic pain. The simple question: Are you troubled by pain? might be sufficient to identify people with a problem. But to ascertain the degree of suffering, individuals would need to be asked to grade their pain, such as mild, moderate, or severe. But neither of these approaches would be sensitive to changes in the degree of pain. This would involve collecting a more detailed gradation of pain so that small changes could be detected. Alternatively, the patient could be asked directly whether their pain had improved or worsened. This example illustrates the distinction between identifying whether patients have a specific symptom, assessing the severity of that symptom and detecting changes in severity over time.

Depending on the purposes of the study, different types of questions will be required to provide sufficient sensitivity.

Cheapness and Ease of Use

The foregoing discussion has highlighted the issues involved in deciding how best to measure the chosen data items. Often there will be several ways of measuring an item, and these will vary in their validity, reliability and sensitivity to change. The differing measures are also likely to vary in the cost of collection and in their difficulty of use. Higher quality measures usually cost more. Thus some consideration should be given to whether the additional cost and difficulty are warranted. Detailed high quality measures are not always needed. Instead, the measure most appropriate to the purposes of the study should be selected.

SELECT THE BEST METHOD OF COLLECTING

Once the list of data items to be collected has been compiled, the best method of collecting them needs to be decided. Data items can be obtained from a variety of sources. These alternative approaches vary in the ease with which they can be used, and the quality of the information which they provide. Thus it is worth reviewing the following:

- abstracting from records
- prospective recording
- interviews and questionnaires
- observational methods of data collection

Abstracting from Records

Health services abound with paper and electronic records of patient information. Casenotes are a commonly used and valuable source of data, particularly of symptoms, diagnosis and treatment. One illustration of this is the study of the prevalence of childhood asthma, based on material recorded in casenotes held by general practitioners (18). It found that, of the children's records reviewed, 24% had symptoms of bronchospasm or wheeze, 8% had a diagnosis of asthma and 5% had had a prescription for anti-asthma medication in the three-month period prior to review.

Casenotes have limitations: they will sometimes not contain all the data required for a research study. Many features of patients and their

Table 13.1   Sources of recorded data

Laboratory records
- pathology
- microbiology
- radiography

Departmental records
- pharmacy
- physiotherapy
- speech therapy
- clinical psychology
- pain clinic

Routinely produced data
- ward computers
- discharge letters
- hospital discharge returns
- cancer registries

General practice
- casenotes
- chronic disease registers
- repeat prescribing registers

management will not be recorded, especially the significant negatives (the results of investigations where the absence of abnormal findings are important for diagnosis and management). This absence of vital items of data has been described as '*the hobgoblin of research that relies on using medical records*' (19). Fortunately, there is a variety of other sources from which data can be obtained, and examples of these are listed in Table 13.1. Computerised records are usually the most easily accessed, and are particularly valuable when large numbers of records need to be reviewed. For example, an investigation of possible discrimination against women in the provision of coronary artery surgery investigated the management of 24 000 patients discharged from hospital with a diagnosis of coronary heart disease (20). It showed that men were significantly more likely than women to undergo revascularisation surgery, an effect seen in two separate regional health authorities.

When information will be contained in more than one source, the guiding principle for the collection of data is to pick the source that will give reliable information most easily. For example, laboratory services can be the easiest way to determine which patients had particular investigations, and what the findings were. Similarly, the easiest way to identify the patients who have been referred to specialist services can be to contact those services directly. Many research studies can be completed using routinely collected data. Often, however, recorded data will be insufficient for research, and new data will need to be collected.

Prospective Recording

When essential data items are nowhere recorded it may be necessary to collect them prospectively on each patient seen. This approach was used to study the safety and value of fibreoptic bronchoscopy in an intensive care unit (21). The study required extensive information on the indications for the procedure, the technical details of how it was performed, the findings of the investigation, and the complications which resulted. The technique was found to be safe and to provide valuable diagnostic information. Prospective recording was required because accurate detailed information were unlikely to be recorded consistently in casenotes, and the staff would be unlikely to remember exactly what happened. When extensive or technical information is required, it will usually have to be specially recorded. Prospective data recording usually involves the completion of a study record during patient management. Study records, like questionnaires, need to be compiled with some care. These design considerations are outlined in the following section.

Interviews and Questionnaires

The most commonly used methods for data collection are personal interview and postal questionnaire. The relative merits of these two techniques are compared in Table 13.2. Interviews are thought to be

Table 13.2 A comparison of postal questionnaires and face-to-face interviews

Postal questionnaires	Interviews
Large numbers can be covered quickly	Fewer people (unless several interviewers used)
Limited amount of data can be collected	Opportunity to probe in depth
Questions can be misunderstood	Interviewer can clarify questions
Questions in fixed sequence	Question sequence can be varied to suit interviewee
Limited opportunity to omit irrelevant questions	Questions can be left out if inappropriate
Allows anonymity	Not anonymous, although interviewer can give reassurance
Cheap	Expensive

better for collecting sensitive personal information, because the interviewer can establish a rapport with the subject. Certainly, personal contact means that answers can often be obtained from individuals who would choose not to return a questionnaire. Interviewers can also be flexible, they can explain when questions are not understood, and can make several attempts to obtain key facts. However, they are much more expensive than written questionnaires. Thus while a researcher might interview seven or eight people in one day, two or three hundred postal questionnaires could be dispatched in the same time.

The construction of questionnaires is one of those tasks which can appear straightforward, but which in practice is difficult to do well. Questions which appear simple to the researcher may perplex the respondents or produce unintelligible responses. The following sequence of steps will help in questionnaire design:

- look for established questionnaires
- formulate the questions
- review the wording
- review the layout
- pilot and revise

Look for Established Questionnaires

There are many established questionnaires which can be used in health services research. The advantage of these is that they can be taken off the shelf, saving a substantial amount of time and effort. They will have been field tested and many will have had their validity, reliability and sensitivity assessed. A variety of measures of quality of life and psychiatric illness have been reviewed in two recent books (4, 5). Another book has reviewed disease-specific measures of quality of life (22). In addition, there will be many other types of questionnaires which will be described only in medical journals. Thus it is worth looking out for them while conducting the literature review.

Formulate the Questions

If there are no suitable established questionnaires, then one will have to be devised. This will involve formulating questions for each of the data items to be collected. Designing these questions should be greatly simplified if it has been clarified exactly what information is wanted.

Questions can be of two types: closed or open-ended. Closed questions ask participants to choose between a set list of items. For example, when asked about symptoms following an operation the respondents might have to choose from a list including pain, nausea, giddiness, cramp, and fever. Providing a list of options makes it easier to answer the questions. However, this runs the risk of prompting respondents to select one answer, even if none applies. Providing a category 'other' with space to specify what it is can partly overcome this problem.

Closed questions simplify the processing of data. The list of possible options can be specified, and the respondents could be asked to tick the appropriate box. A code can be placed next to each box for data entry. For example, when enquiring about marital status the options offered would be:

Marital status
   single   ☐   1
   cohabiting/married   ☐   2
   separated   ☐   3
   widowed   ☐   4
   divorced   ☐   5

Open questions are of the form: What symptoms did you have following the treatment? They allow the respondent to give any response they wish. Thus open-ended questions allow issues to be probed, revealing responses which the researcher might never have imagined. But these questions generate additional work at the stage of data processing. To be analysed by computer the various responses have to be given numerical codes. This can be a tedious task if there are more than a handful of forms to be processed. Open questions are often used in exploratory or pilot work, where the intention is to identify the list of options to be used in closed questions.

Review the Wording

Once the questions have been formulated they need to be reviewed so that ambiguities and difficult terms or phrases can be corrected. It is surprisingly difficult to compose questions which are readily understood. Some of the commonly encountered problems, together with examples of how to circumvent them, are shown in Table 13.3. When reviewed many of the flaws are readily apparent, but some might well be overlooked. A useful approach to identifying these types of problem is to ask of each question: If I really wanted to misinterpret this question, which part of it would I choose to misunderstand?

Table 13.3 Problems of question phrasing

Problems	Examples	Solutions
Technical terms (especially to patients)	*Have you heard of laparoscopic surgery?*	Rephrase to use lay terms, e.g. *Have you heard about keyhole surgery?*
Leading questions	*How often do your children brush their teeth?*	Rephrase, e.g. *Do your children brush their teeth?*
Composite questions	*Was the doctor ever inattentive or uncaring?*	Split into separate questions
Double negatives	*Would you not have preferred to have not been asked?*	Disentangle, e.g. *Would you have preferred not to have been asked?*
Presuming questions	*How long have you smoked cigarettes?*	Use filter question first, e.g. *Do you smoke?*
Prestige questions	*Does the treatment cause you to pass wind?*	Defuse by rephrasing, e.g. *This treatment causes some patients to pass wind, does this ever happen to you?*
Imprecise questions	*Are you usually seen quickly?*	Be specific, e.g. *Have you ever had to wait more than 30 minutes?*
Words open to interpretation	*Is the result what you expected?*	Be specific, e.g. *Did you expect a positive result to the pregnancy test?*

Review the Layout

Whether a questionnaire is sent by post or used in an interview, it has to be both intelligible and interesting to the respondent. Thus it is essential that the questions are arranged in a sequence which appears logical and is easy to follow. Not doing this may antagonise the respondent. The first question should be simple to answer and should be the kind of question people would expect, given the stated purposes of the study. Questions which cover related items can be grouped together. It is often recommended that potentially difficult or embarrassing questions should be put towards the end of the sequence.

When questionnaires are to be completed by respondents, they should be visually attractive and easy to follow. This may only involve having a space between succeeding questions and indenting lines when there is more than one part to the question. Poorly laid out questions will affect the quality of data collected and may discourage some people from completing the questionnaire.

The layout should also simplify the task of coding and processing the data. For example, if the written answers are scattered across a page, some may be missed when the data are being input into a computer. It is helpful if answers are aligned vertically so the eye can easily follow them. If this cannot be easily achieved a right hand margin (labelled 'for office use only') could be provided so that all the answers can be transcribed into it. A small investment to achieve a helpful layout can save a great deal of effort when it comes to processing the collected data.

Pilot and Revise

Despite close attention to their design, questionnaires will always contain flaws which the researcher cannot see. Those attracted to conspiracy theory might think that there is a malign spirit of questionnaire design, who surreptitiously inserts ambiguities and confusions. The truth is more likely that the researcher is too intimately involved with the questionnaire to see its problems. Whatever the explanation, the only way to eradicate the flaws is to try the questionnaire out on a small group prior to its use in the main study. This group should be similar to the group who are to be studied. Little would be gained by trying out on colleagues a questionnaire designed for the general public. Groups with specialist knowledge will understand technical terms that the general public will not, and because they know how the health service works they may correctly interpret a question which lay people might find confusing. Piloting is essential: unpiloted questionnaires are a recipe for disaster.

Observational Methods of Data Collection

Interviews and self-completed questionnaires are flexible tools which can be used in a wide variety of situations, but their pervasiveness may inhibit the use of other methods. In many instances neither of these methods would be appropriate. For example, in a study of the quality of care given to patients dying in hospital, the use of questionnaires and interviews with the staff could have been misleading. The method which was employed, direct observation, revealed many inadequacies in care: *'oral hygiene was often poor, thirst remained unquenched, and little assistance was given to encourage eating'* (23). It is most likely that the staff involved were unaware of these deficiencies, and would not have reported them when asked.

Observational methods will be particularly useful when the focus of the study lies with subtle features of the process of care which are unlikely to be recorded or readily apparent to staff. For example, when it was found that 45% of central venous catheters had to be removed because of sepsis, the staff inserting the catheters were closely observed (24). One of the main contributors to the occurrence of sepsis was poor hand-washing technique, particularly by junior medical staff on rotation. This finding would not have been uncovered through interview or casenote review.

When observational techniques are to be used, it is important to recognise that they are still a method of conducting a survey. There may be a tendency just to observe those individuals who happen to be on hand. The unspoken justification, that one is only having a look, is not satisfactory. Instead, care needs to be taken that an atypical sample is not obtained, otherwise misleading results may be obtained. An observational approach to research does not relieve the researcher of the burden of considering the issues involved in survey design (see Chapter 6).

Reviewing the Methods

The variety of possible methods of data collection poses the question of which to use for a particular study. The method will usually be evident if the research question has been refined and a list has been made of the required data items. When there is doubt about which methods should be used, it can be resolved by asking of each potential source of data whether it is likely to provide complete and accurate information. If more than one method meets these requirements, then choose the one which will be cheapest and easiest to use. More commonly all the possible methods will have some defects. Then it becomes a case of choosing the method which will give sufficiently high quality data without costing too much. Research is a pragmatic business, and studies are never entirely free from error.

Sometimes it may not be obvious where the necessary information will be located, nor which will be the easiest source to use. The answer is to have a look, to conduct a small pilot study to resolve the problem. The accuracy of the data in different sources is sometimes surprising. A recent study compared the accuracy of casenotes versus interview on obstetric and contraceptive history (26). Although some items were not recorded in the notes, the conclusion was that they could have been used successfully and *'response rates would have been higher, recall bias eliminated, and the cost of the study halved'*.

In some studies more than one method will need to be used. For example, a study of the reasons for some pregnant women being susceptible to rubella infection used personal interviews, postal questionnaires to general practitioners, casenotes and laboratory records (25). The reasons uncovered were a mixture of non-vaccination and apparently failed vaccination, but fortunately almost all received rubella vaccination postpartum. Multiple sources of data will often be needed when the process of care is being investigated and direct observational techniques cannot be used.

DRAW UP THE CODING SCHEDULE

When a data set consists of a few items collected on a handful of patients, it may be possible to do the analysis by hand. In all other circumstances the data will have to be entered into a computer for analysis. This places several requirements on the coding and organisation of the data so that it is suitable for analysis. These are:

- allocate subject identifier
- ensure fixed sequence
- use numerical codes
- decide coding conventions
- avoid free text

Allocate Subject Identifier

Conventionally the first item in each record is a unique serial number, avoiding the need for names and addresses to be held on computer. The serial number can then form the link between the computer record and the original document. This makes it possible to check back to the original data sources should the need arise. There are often occasions during the analysis that unusual values are encountered, and the researcher may wish to check against the source document.

Ensure Fixed Sequence

Computers need the data for each subject to be entered in exactly the same way. Table 13.4 illustrates the layout suitable for computer analysis. The data for each subject (be it patient, health care professional or emergency trolley) is laid out along a row. The items should be arranged in a fixed sequence so that, for example, age is always the second item and disease duration the fifth. The computer can locate variables by their position, and will get confused if their positions vary. (More sophisticated methods of storing data are available using relational databases. But these are seldom needed in well-focused studies. Simple data organisation has much to commend it.)

Use Numerical Codes

The endpoint of data processing is to have a list of data items in the form of numerical codes. Closed questions can allocate the codes 1, 2, 3 . . . up to the maximum number of alternatives. Thus, instead of recording sex as male or female it is coded 1 (=male) or 2 (=female). It would be possible to code this item as M or F, but there are many situations in which the computer needs the codes in numeric form, so it is usually best to start with them in this form. The requirement for numerically coded data means that information on items such as disease severity has to be collected in a way that can be easily reduced to a limited number of numerical categories.

Decide Coding Conventions

It can be useful to adopt some coding conventions. Questions with yes/ no answers could always be coded yes =1, no = 2. Otherwise if there were several yes/no questions there could be confusion about which code to use. A specific code can also be used to indicate that a data item was not recorded, commonly 9 (or 99, or 999 as appropriate) are used. Having a code for missing items is one instance of ensuring that there are codes for all eventualities. Leaving a blank on the data form runs the risk of all items after the blank being moved one place along, with disastrous consequences for data analysis. Thus codes could be provided for items which are not relevant to selected individuals (e.g. when asking a man about the number of completed pregnancies). They could also be used for not known (e.g. to indicate that a subject could not recall the nature of their previous treatment).

Table 13.4 Layout of data for entry into a computer

Serial number	Age	Sex	Supervising doctor	Disease duration	Symptom 1 score	Symptom 2 score	Disease severity	No. of complications
1	45	2	5	14	3	2	3	1
2	38	2	4	12	1	1	1	3
3	69	1	1	59	4	5	5	12
–	–	–	–	–	–	–	–	–
–	–	–	–	–	–	–	–	–
–	–	–	–	–	–	–	–	–
73	26	1	4	3	1	1	1	0

Avoid Free Text

Sometimes it may be difficult to derive a suitable coding scheme and it may be tempting to postpone this activity, by entering the data as free text (plain English). The problem is that when stored in this form the data are much more difficult to analyse. The hope that they will be converted to numerical codes at some future date is misplaced. If the data are not coded at entry they will almost certainly never be analysed.

COMMENT AND FURTHER READING

Collecting data is at the heart of research. Sadly it is one activity whose planning receives far less attention than it deserves. There is a tendency to begin data collection prematurely, before the data items and their measurement have been properly described. It may be that, as the excitement of developing the research idea has faded, there is insufficient resolve to sort out the nuts and bolts of which data items to collect and how best to collect them. But the success of any study really does hang on whether the appropriate items have been collected correctly. There is no alternative to working painstakingly through the activities described in this chapter.

There are three good textbooks devoted to the design and use of questionnaires (27–29). In describing these processes they also touch on many of the issues of deciding which data to collect and selecting the best method of collecting them. These books vary in the emphasis and approach which they take, and it could be worth taking a look at more than one of them.

REFERENCES

1. Abramson, JH. *Survey Methods in Community Medicine: Epidemiological Studies, Programme Evaluation, Clinical Trials* 4th edn. Edinburgh: Churchill Livingstone, 1990.
2. Jenkinson, D. Natural course of 500 consecutive cases of whooping cough: a general practice population study. *British Medical Journal* 1995; **310**: 299–302.
3. Fitzpatrick, R. Surveys of patient satisfaction: I—Important general considerations. *British Medical Journal* 1991; **302**: 887–9.
4. Bowling, A. *Measuring Health: A Review of Quality of Life Measurement Scales.* Buckingham: Open University Press, 1991.
5. Wilkin, D, Hallam, L and Doggett, M. *Measures of Need and Outcome for Primary Health Care.* Oxford: Oxford University Press, 1992.

6. Leete, R and Fox, J. Registrar General's social classes: origins and uses. *Population Trends* 1977; **8**: 1–7.

7. Liberatos, P, Link, BG and Kelsey, JL. The measurement of social class in epidemiology. *Epidemiologic Reviews* 1988; **10**: 87–121.

8. Probert, CJS, Emmett, PM and Heaton, KW. Intestinal transit time in the population calculated from self made observations of defecation. *Journal of Epidemiology and Community Health* 1993; **47**: 331–3.

9. Doyle, D. Morphine: myths, morality and economics. *Postgraduate Medical Journal* 1991; **67** (Supplement 2): S70–3.

10. Scully, C, Porter, S and Greenman, J. What to do about halitosis [editorial]. *British Medical Journal* 1994; **308**: 217–18.

11. Atherton, JC and Spiller, RC. The urea breath test for *Helicobacter pylori*. *Gut* 1994; **35**: 723–5.

12. Jarvis, MJ, Russell, MAH, Feyerabend, C, Eiser, JR and Morgan, M. Passive exposure to tobacco smoke: saliva cotinine concentrations in a representative population sample of non-smoking schoolchildren. *British Medical Journal* 1985; **291**: 927–9.

13. Prineas, RJ. *Blood Pressure Sounds: Their Measurement and Meaning. A Training Manual*. Minneapolis: Gamma Medical Products Corporation, 1978.

14. Feinstein, AR. A bibliography of publications on observer variability. *Journal of Chronic Diseases* 1985; **38**(8): 619–32.

15. Langer, LM, Zimmerman, RS and Cabral, RJ. Perceived versus actual condom skills among clients at sexually transmitted disease clinics. *Public Health Reports* 1994; **109**(5): 683–7.

16. Portney, LG and Watkins, MP. *Foundations of Clinical Research: Applications to Practice*. Norwalk: Appleton & Lange, 1993.

17. Goldberg, D, Bridges, K, Duncan-Jones, P and Grayson, D. Detecting anxiety and depression in general medical settings. *British Medical Journal* 1988; **297**: 897–9.

18. Neville, RG, Bryce, FP, Robertson, FM, Crombie, IK and Clark, RA. Diagnosis and treatment of asthma in children: usefulness of a review of medical records. *British Journal of General Practice* 1992; **42**: 501–3.

19. Gehlbach, SH. *Interpreting the Medical Literature* 3rd edn. New York: McGraw-Hill, 1993: p33.

20. Petticrew, M, McKee, M and Jones, J. Coronary artery surgery: are women discriminated against? *British Medical Journal* 1993; **306**: 1164–6.

21. Turner, JS, Willcox, PA, Hayhurst, MD and Potgieter, PD. Fiberoptic bronchoscopy in the intensive care unit—a prospective study of 147 procedures in 107 patients. *Critical Care Medicine* 1994; **22**(2): 259–64.

22. Bowling, A. *Measuring Disease: A Review of Disease-Specific Quality of Life Measurement Scales*. Buckingham: Open University Press, 1995.

23. Mills, M, Davies, HTO and Macrae, WA. Care of dying patients in hospital. *British Medical Journal* 1994; **309**: 583–6.

24. Puntis, JWL, Holden, CE, Smallman, S, Finkel, Y, George, RH and Booth, IW. Staff training: a key factor in reducing intravascular catheter sepsis. *Archives of Disease in Childhood* 1990; **65**: 335–7.

25. Lawman, S, Morton, K and Best, JM. Reasons for rubella susceptibility among pregnant women in West Lambeth. *Journal of the Royal Society of Medicine* 1994; **87**: 263–4.

26. Chilvers, CED, Pike, MC, Taylor, CN, *et al.* General practitioner notes as a

source of information for case-control studies in young women. *Journal of Epidemiology and Community Health* 1994; **48**: 92–7.

27. Bennett, AE and Ritchie, K. *Questionnaires in Medicine: A Guide to Their Design and Use*. London: Oxford University Press, 1975.

28. Oppenheim, AN. *Questionnaire Design, Interviewing and Attitude Measurement* 2nd edn. London: Pinter Publishers, 1992.

29. Streiner, DL and Norman, GR. *Health Measurement Scales: A Practical Guide to their Development and Use*. Oxford: Oxford University Press, 1989.

Chapter 14

PRACTICAL ISSUES IN THE DESIGN AND CONDUCT OF STUDIES

The previous chapters have shown how research questions are fashioned, and have described the research methods which can be used to answer them. But they have not dealt with the many practical issues of designing and running a research project. These arise whatever the research method being used, and are outlined in this chapter.

BEGINNING THE PROCESS

The process of designing a study can be one of the most enjoyable stages of research. There are a series of problems to be solved, and the researcher can sit in a chair and ponder them (or walk in the fresh air if that stimulates the brain). Many are best solved in brainstorming sessions with colleagues. The design can be thought of as a two-stage process. An initial broad outline is prepared and reviewed before the detailed design is constructed.

The Importance of Planning

A central theme of this book is the importance of planning when carrying out research. There is often an almost irresistible urge to get the study underway as soon as possible, often before the design has been properly worked out. It is easy to collect data, the trick is in obtaining useful data. Having a large number of measurements on a large group of patients does not mean that anything useful will be contained in them. It is only when the purpose of the data collection is clearly stated, and the data items carefully selected, that meaningful results will be obtained.

Premature data collection is one instance of confusing activity with progress. This confusion is summed up in the old saying: *'what is the use of running when you are on the wrong road?'* Planning begins by asking a series of questions:

- What exactly do I want to do?
- How do I do it?
- Can I do it?
- Is it worth doing?
- Has it been done before?

Only when all these questions have been considered in some depth can the study begin in earnest. Study design takes the answers to these questions and crafts them into a detailed plan of action.

State the Initial Design

The questions on planning form the prelude to the development of the study design. Taking this forward involves three activities:

- define the research question
- select the research method
- specify the data to be collected

The detail of the research design is driven by the exact nature of the research question. Thus the research question needs to be reviewed, appraised and recast until it is fully worked out. Techniques for doing this are described in Chapter 3. The development of a researchable question leads directly to the specification of the most appropriate research method. The research methods were reviewed in Chapters 6 to 10, and techniques for selecting the most appropriate were reviewed in Chapter 11. Having decided on the method, attention focuses on the data needed to answer the question. The issues of data collection were reviewed in Chapter 13.

The development of the research design is commonly presented (as here) as if the stages are carried out in sequence. In practice, the design of research is less a matter of following a straight path than of going round in circles. Decisions on some points of the design may require modifications to other parts which had been decided on previously. The best approach is to have an initial stab at each of the three activities, then set about developing each in more depth.

Table 14.1 Activities where specialist advice might be needed

Activity	Specialist
Sample size, methods of analysis	Statistician
Measuring beliefs, attitudes, behaviour	Medical sociologist, health psychologist
Assessing costs of care, and costs of disability	Health economist
Describing flows of patients through health care, predicting future health care demands	Operations researcher
Developing questionnaires, developing study design	Experienced researcher
Developing patient information leaflet	Health promotion specialist

Decide about Specialist Advice

As the design evolves, it will gradually become clear when specialist advice is necessary. Table 14.1 lists the types of activity where advice may be needed, and the corresponding specialist. It is important to seek advice early in the development of the design, as this may influence key aspects of the study. Statisticians, in particular, lament being approached at a late stage in the study, usually after the data have been collected, in the hope that they can make up for deficiencies in the design: *'one of the saddest aspects of being a statistician is being unable to rescue a poorly designed study by pulling a magical statistical analysis out of the hat'* (1).

When approaching other professionals for advice, it is important to recognise that the specialist must also benefit from the encounter. In days gone by advice was freely given, as part of the regular duties of a researcher. But in these days of professional assessment, researchers can ill afford to dispense free advice. Most professionals will willingly give up the odd half-hour with no thought of reward. But when it comes to substantial input, the kind which is often needed, appropriate academic credit should be given. The specialist should be an acknowledged collaborator, and named on grant applications and papers. If their advice is worth seeking out, then their contribution needs to be fully recognised.

DEVELOPING THE DESIGN

The initial design provides an outline of the research method and data to be collected. But before the study is begun the fine details need to be worked out. This involves more than simply clarifying exactly what will be done and how it will be done. The steps to be followed are:

- write the protocol
- obtain ethical approval
- obtain funding
- inform interested parties
- register under the Data Protection Act
- develop the data processing
- pilot all the stages
- review the design

Write the Protocol

A useful way to develop the detailed design is by writing a study protocol. All research studies will benefit from having a protocol formally written out. Protocols need not be lengthy, detailed documents that take weeks to write. For simple studies it may take no more than an afternoon to compose a satisfactory protocol. The important point is that one has been written. The act of writing focuses the mind, and highlights aspects of the design which are much less well defined than had previously been thought. It is far better to identify defects at an early stage, than to discover halfway through a project that no one is clear what they are supposed to be doing. The protocol can be divided into a number of stages.

Background

The background, or introduction, sets the scene for the proposed study. It briefly describes previous work in the area, and outlines the gaps in knowledge which require further research. It is not necessary to provide a comprehensive review of the literature. Instead, this section should explain why there is an urgent need for the new study.

Aims

The aims of the study should be set out clearly and briefly. The aims will follow from the gaps in knowledge identified in the Background. They will frequently be cast as questions that the study is seeking to answer.

Method

This section describes the particular research method to be used and should outline why it will fulfil the study aims. It will state where the study will be conducted, and how the subjects are to be obtained. The exact nature of the group to be studied should be described and, if appropriate, how informed consent is to be obtained. The required data items should be specified together with an indication of how they are to be collected. If standard questionnaires or measuring techniques are to be used, they should be referenced. The statistical techniques should also be listed. The Methods section should demonstrate that the study is feasible and scientifically rigorous.

Sample Size

A sample size calculation is, strictly speaking, a part of the Methods section. But it is marked out separately because it is essential for any research study. If the study is too small it will fail to provide an answer to the research question; if it is too large it will consume time and resources which could be better spent elsewhere. The issue of sample size was dealt with for the various research methods in Chapters 6 to 9.

Resources

The resources for research cover materials, equipment and staff. They include envelopes, stamps, photocopying, travel and staff time for data collection, processing and analysis. One resource which is sometimes overlooked is the time required to monitor study progress and supervise junior staff doing the day-to-day work. Underestimating the resources required can be embarrassing, often resulting in fewer subjects being recruited than was intended. But underfunding can also be catastrophic: if, for example, there were insufficient funds to pay for the postage for questionnaires, or to pay a data clerk to process the returned forms. Thus it is best, if an error is to be made, to slightly overestimate costs. If external funding is being sought, a small increase in the total cost is unlikely to affect the likelihood of a grant being awarded (providing the details of the costing appear reasonable).

Plan

The plan of the study is really the timetable according to which the project will be carried out. This may include a development phase, during which questionnaires and other materials are designed and tested. It is helpful if the plan details what should be achieved at regular intervals throughout the study. For example, a nine-month study should list the activities to be completed at least every month: during the early phases when the study is being set up it might be necessary to specify activities on a weekly basis.

Writing the study protocol should lead to a greatly clarified design. It should also indicate the feasibility of the project, given the constraints of time and resources.

Obtain Ethical Approval

The paramount importance of ethical issues in research was described in Chapter 1. Research studies carried out within the NHS will almost always require approval from an ethical committee. Even if you think a research study probably does not need ethical approval, it is best to proceed as if it did, and seek advice from the local ethical committee at an early stage.

Applications for ethical approval are considered by local research ethics committees (LRECs). These are organised on a health authority basis. LRECs have 8 to 12 members, comprising hospital doctors and GPs, nurses, scientists and at least two laypersons. They are unpaid, but the task they perform is onerous and carries with it a great deal of responsibility. Many ethical committees have a standard form to be completed, which should be submitted in addition to the detailed study protocol. When planning an application it can be helpful to make an informal approach to the LREC, possibly through the secretary, to see what advice they would offer.

LRECs will be concerned with the scientific merits of the study and, most importantly, with the effect which the research may have on those taking part. They will want to be assured that there is no pressure, financial or other, on individuals to take part. One of the overriding concerns of ethical committees is with informed consent. The Declaration of Helsinki has as one of its principles that 'In any research on human beings, each potential subject must be adequately informed of the aims, methods, anticipated benefits and potential hazards of the study and the discomfort it may entail' (2). The need for informed consent is emphasised in the guidelines on ethics which have recently been reissued by the Medical Research Council and many of the Royal Colleges.

Informed consent is a complex matter. Participants should have the purposes of the study explained to them and be given a description of how it will affect them. This must include an account of any risks associated with the research, should these exist. Participants must know that involvement in the research is entirely voluntary and that they can leave the study at any time. If they are patients they must be told that their treatment will not be influenced by whether they take part or not. Participants must also be given an information leaflet which contains the same information, but which they can take away with them to think about afterwards. The intention of the process is that potential participants can come to a balanced decision about whether they wish to take part.

Obtaining informed consent is not just a matter for adults. Young persons over the age of 16 years are considered capable of deciding for themselves whether to participate in research (2). Younger children are also considered capable of giving valid consent, if their medical practitioner thinks they can understand what the research involves and what consequences it may have. In practice a lower limit will be set by whether the child can read the information leaflet and consent form. Whatever the age of the child, it is important to be sure that they truly understand what is being proposed: *'it is advisable for the qualified medical practitioner to be satisfied that the child has a greater level of understanding than is necessary'* (2).

The other issue which taxes ethical committees is whether participants may be at any risk from the research. Risk may result from the procedures carried out during the research, or even from information given during the process of obtaining informed consent. The task of the LREC is to ensure that any risk is small enough to be acceptable. At first sight it might appear that no risk would be acceptable. But the view taken is that there needs to be a balance between the risk to the individual and the potential benefits from the research to society as a whole. It is argued that so long as the risk is minimal, then worthwhile research should be permitted. Clearly these are very difficult issues to resolve, balancing risks against benefits. There are many books which address these ethical concerns in more detail. One particularly lucid and thorough book was produced by the British Medical Association (3), but texts by Garrett and colleagues (4) and Johnson (5) are also informative.

Obtain Funding

Research costs money, and it will often be necessary to seek some form of funding. The discipline of writing the protocol should have indicated whether additional funds will be needed to complete the study. Obtaining funding often appears daunting, yet it need not be. It can be approached in the same step-by-step way that the study design was developed. The stages in obtaining funding are:

- identify potential funding bodies
- clarify research interests
- follow the application guidelines
- ensure clarity
- emphasise the implications
- keep on trying

Identify Potential Funding Bodies

There are a large number of organisations which support research. Local sources of funding include local charities who have an interest in research and health trusts who may have endowment funds. Many district health authorities will have research budgets. The regional health authorities have research managers whose role is to advise and encourage those wishing to conduct research. They will have details of all the local funding bodies as well as the national ones.

Much medical research is funded by charities. Some charities focus on particular diseases, such as the National Asthma Campaign and the Arthritis and Rheumatism Council. Others, such as the Wellcome Trust and the Nuffield Foundation, cover a wider array of topics. The charities also vary in the sums which they have available for research: some can provide only modest amounts, whereas others spend millions of pounds each year. The addresses and interests of these charities are reviewed annually in *The Association of Medical Research Charities Handbook*. Copies of this handbook can be obtained from:

> The Association of Medical Research Charities
> 29–35 Farringdon Road
> London EC1M 3JB

The Medical Research Council (MRC) plays a major role in funding health services research. It will fund small project grants, up to £30 000, as well as much larger grants of the order of several hundred thousand pounds. Small projects will receive much quicker decisions on funding than larger projects. The evaluation process of the latter can take up to a year, so that early planning is essential. Further information about the MRC's role in supporting health services research can be obtained from:

Dr A C Peatfield
Secretary, Health Services and Public Health Research Board
Medical Research Council
20 Park Crescent
London W1N 4AL

The government, through the Department of Health in England (and equivalent bodies in Scotland, Northern Ireland and Wales) also disburses funds for health services research. Addresses can be obtained from:

Research and Development Division
Department of Health
Room 449
Richmond House
79 Whitehall
London SW1A 2NS

Clarify Research Interests

Funding bodies have widely different research interests. Even those which have what appears a broad remit will have specialist areas which they regard as high priority, and others in which they have little interest. It is likely that a given research study will be thought of more highly by some funding bodies than others.

The funding bodies usually publish their areas of interest. In addition, many of them can be approached for informal discussions about proposed research studies. This will clarify the types of research study which they are interested in funding within their priority areas. It is often possible to change the emphases in a protocol so that the aims more closely fit the interests of the funding body.

Follow the Application Guidelines

Funding bodies also vary in their requirements for a grant application. These requirements are usually stated in the documents which accompany the application form and it is important to read them carefully. Some bodies require a two-stage application process. A brief outline of the project is first assessed and, if this is judged satisfactory, a more detailed application is requested. Most funding bodies require a detailed protocol, usually in the form outlined above, although there will usually be variations on the theme. One additional section which is often requested is a justification of the money requested.

Applications also ask what resources and facilities are already available. These may include anything from computers and software to desks and filing cabinets. The intention is to show that the funding body is paying for only a part of the total: that they are getting much more than they are paying for.

Ensure Clarity

It sometimes seems to researchers that funding bodies are almost wilful in the ways they choose to misunderstand perfectly clear grant applications. More likely, the researcher is simply too familiar with the ideas to be able to recognise ambiguities in the application. When assessing the application the funding body will ask the following questions:

- Is it an important research question?
- Is the method appropriate and fully described?
- Do the applicants have the expertise?
- Can it be done in the allotted time?
- Are the resources requested appropriate?

Thus care needs to be taken that the answers to these questions emerge clearly from the application. The Aims section should be short and snappy. The Methods should demonstrate that the applicants really know how to carry out the study. But above all, the implications of the research need to be emphasised.

Emphasise the Implications

The most important part of a research study is the potential implications of the findings. All funding bodies want to be recognised as the organisation behind the major breakthrough that transformed health care. And rightly so. Trivial research is of little interest to anyone. Thus the researcher needs to demonstrate why the findings could be important: how they have much wider implications than the local circumstances of the study. The art of writing grant applications is to make the proposed study appear central to a host of possible developments. The idea is to make it clear that the findings from this study will reverberate across health care.

Keep on Trying

Success in obtaining funding is not guaranteed, even with very high quality applications. Even experienced researchers expect to have some of their applications turned down. If an application is rejected, this is not final; it does not signal the end of a project. There are other funding bodies which can be tried. Funding bodies are composed of a set of individuals with their own preferences. It can easily happen that one committee may reject an application, while another may really like it.

The not insubstantial chance of rejection should also temper the amount of effort put into preparing the application. Applications need to be of a high standard, as poorly thought out, badly prepared applications will not be funded. But the effort should be limited by what is called the eighty:twenty rule. This holds that for any task 80% can be completed fairly quickly (20% of the effort). But the remaining 20% of the task requires very much more work (80% of the effort). The implication of this rule is that several good applications could be prepared in the time which it takes to produce one of supremely high quality.

In general, if the research idea is a good one (with substantial implications), and it looks as though the study is feasible, there is a good chance of funding. However, no application will be perfect. If the funding body is interested in the research but has concerns about specific details of the application, it is likely to ask for clarification or modification of these. The researcher will then be given the opportunity to modify and resubmit the application.

Inform Interested Parties

Research can have implications for health care professionals other than those involved directly in a study. People rightly want to know about research going on locally, and some will be offended if they are not informed. Thus it is worth thinking around a project to try to identify who might be interested in knowing that a study is underway.

A variety of individuals and institutions may need to be contacted. If the research is conducted within a health trust it is advisable to inform the trust authorities. Most areas will have a research coordinator or research manager, who can advise on local procedures. This may include entering the project into the local research register. Sometimes it may be mandatory to obtain official permission before undertaking a study. For example, before contacting GPs for permission to send questionnaires to their patients, it is essential to have obtained the approval of the local GP subcommittee. In other instances it is a simple matter of courtesy to inform senior staff. If the research could be relevant to nurses, or pharmacists, or dietitians, then the local leaders of the appropriate professional groups could be contacted. Keeping people informed helps to keep them on side.

Register under the Data Protection Act

In 1984 the Data Protection Act came onto statute (6). Its primary aim was to protect individuals against the misuse of data held on computer. Although the emphasis was on personal and financial information, the Act also covers data gathered during medical research. It requires that the existence of data on individuals which is kept on a computer be registered. Registration involves the completion of a form, stating the types of data held, the uses to which these will be put, and the individuals who have access to it. Many institutions have a data protection officer who will supply and deal with the necessary forms. It is extremely unlikely that any untoward events will occur as a result of holding data on a computer. But as registration is such a simple process, it is best to follow it (and it is a legal requirement).

The Office of the Data Protection Registrar could be written to directly at

Springfield House
Water Lane
Wilmslow
Cheshire SK9 5AX

Develop the Data Processing

The best way to handle the processing of data depends largely on the size of the data set. Small amounts of data, say 20 to 30 two-page questionnaires, can probably be keyed in by a secretary or even by the researcher. Larger studies should consider using an experienced data entry clerk, or a data processing unit in a university department. Experienced data processing staff can enter data more quickly and more accurately. As with other stages of the research process, it is helpful to seek advice. Whatever approach is selected for data entry, there are several issues to be considered. These are:

- form handling
- computers
- software for data entry
- verification

- back-up
- counting the forms
- checking selected records

Form Handling

Questionnaires and record forms have a quite amazing propensity to disappear. Even when an apparently foolproof system of form handling and data processing has been established, some forms will manage to avoid inclusion in the final data file. The researcher will have to design a method for the safe distribution and return of forms. The forms received should be numbered so that checks can be carried out during processing to determine whether any are being lost. The process of checking should be carried out regularly during the study, so that any defects in form handling can be quickly remedied.

Computers

Computers are now indispensable to virtually all research studies, the only exceptions being case studies and small case series. The contribution of computers can be immense in terms of the time and effort they save, but this is restricted to some clearly defined tasks. Basically the computer is an idiot which can count and process data with incredible speed. It cannot think or warn the researchers that what it has been told to do makes no sense. Instead it blindly follows instructions, carrying out analyses regardless of whether the data have been inadvertently shuffled during processing. From the researchers' perspective present day computers have one major defect: they lack judgement. Thus the guiding principle when using computers is that the researcher must supply all the judgement and common sense. It is also helpful to assume that if things can go wrong they will, and quite often they will go wrong even when in theory they cannot.

Computers evolve so rapidly that it is possibly unwise for a textbook to give advice on which kind to buy. Fortunately for most research projects the choice of hardware is not critical: any up-to-date, mid-range machine from a reputable company will have sufficient power to process and analyse the data. Buying an older machine can pose problems. It may not have sufficient power to run current versions of software packages. The counsel of the two Ms, modern and middle of the road, is a safe one to follow.

Software for Data Entry

There are basically three types of software package which are commonly used to handle research data: spreadsheets, databases and statistical packages. Spreadsheets are usually easy to use, and organise the data in the type of grid shown in Table 13.4. They are widely used in business and financial departments. Spreadsheets provide a simple means for data entry, but are less suited to data analysis. Although many supply some statistical functions, it is usually much easier to analyse data using a dedicated statistical package. One important feature when choosing a spreadsheet is to ensure that it can write data to a file which can then be read into a statistical package.

Database packages can also be used for data entry. However, they offer many sophisticated data handling techniques which most research projects do not need. They are also restricted in the range of statistical functions which they provide. Thus they are probably best avoided unless there is a need for their specialised features (for example, the ability to cope with patients who make substantially different numbers of follow-up visits). If a database package is to be used for data entry, it is important to ensure that it can export the data for use in a statistical package.

Statistical packages which are used for analysis often provide data entry facilities like those of the spreadsheet. Thus they can be conveniently used for entering small amounts of data. However, some are less useful for entering large data sets, because they do not provide a facility for verification.

Verification

Data entry, like all human activity, is an error-prone process. The trouble with errors in data entry is that the consequence can be disastrous. For example, if digits were transposed then a person aged 19 years would be converted to 91 years. If there were a simple miskeying, then a systolic blood pressure of 110 mm Hg could become 210 mm Hg. To reduce the frequency of errors the data can be entered twice. The two versions are compared and discrepancies resolved by referring to the original document. This process is known as double key verification and can be carried out simply by many computer packages.

Back-up

Whenever data files are created in a computer a second copy, a back-up, should be taken on a floppy disk. (The same is true for documents created with a word processor.) With a back-up it is simple to recover a data file if it is corrupted, or worse deleted, during processing or analysis. The larger the data file the more important taking a back-up becomes because of the cost of re-entering the data. Making a back-up copy on the hard disk is only a partial solution: the computer may break down and lose all the information on the hard disk. Thus files should be regularly copied to separate disks, clearly labelled and securely stored. Most researchers take a back-up copy onto floppy disk after each session in which data have been entered or modified. Many will also take a second back-up on a monthly basis (or when important new data have been added), and store this at a different site. If this seems a bit of a bind, think how much more it would be if a key data file were irretrievably lost. There are only two types of computer user: those who have lost data, and those who have not (yet). Data are expensive to collect and only too easy to lose.

Checking Selected Records

When the data have all been entered it is worth checking a few selected records. Computers may be a boon to data processing and analysis but, through human error, they have the capacity really to foul things up. Thus it is best to make sure that nothing disastrous has happened during processing. One simple check is to take the first and the last records, and two or three others, and check what is in the computer against the original paper document. The records should be in the correct order, and the sequence of data items within them should match the source document. Errors detected by this simple check would be a cause for serious concern.

Pilot all the Stages

One of the characteristics of research is the occurrence of unforeseen difficulties. They always crop up, often in places where nothing should have gone wrong. The researcher has simply to recognise this, and try to minimise the opportunities for disaster. The pilot study is one device to achieve this. All parts of the study should be tried out in advance to check whether they work. It is not enough to review the study design and conclude that it should work; the design needs to be tested. This might mean, for example, contacting some patients, interviewing them, and analysing their responses. If the study involves taking measurements or sending specimens to a laboratory, these stages too should be tested.

The pilot study seeks answers to a number of questions. Can the study subjects be identified and recruited? Can all the measurements be made accurately? Is the questionnaire easily understood and unambiguous? Who will carry out the study activities; when, where and how? What effect will these activities have on professional duties? How will the data be processed and analysed? At the end of the pilot study the researcher should have evidence that all the stages of the study will work. Piloting will not guarantee that a study will be trouble free, but failing to pilot almost certainly spells disaster.

Review the Design

The design of a study needs to be reviewed on a regular basis, asking questions like:

- How good is the research question?
- Is the design fully worked out?
- Have all the flaws been detected?
- Is the study feasible?

These questions should be asked during the development of the design, after the pilot study, and during the conduct of the study. These questions really only identify broad areas of interest. More detailed questions to appraise the study design are given in Table 14.2. All of these questions should have been answered, and attempts made to remedy deficiencies, before the study proper is begun. The alternative is to run the risk of conducting a study which will fail.

Be Realistic

Research studies are never perfect, they all contain flaws and imperfections. Eliminating some flaws might be possible, but it may also be very expensive. There is a trade-off between cost and quality which, consciously or not, is resolved in all projects. The intention is to make the study as good as possible within the available resources. Every effort is made to prevent possible flaws, but without becoming totally obsessed by them. The important thing about flaws is not that they are all eliminated, but that the types which remain are identified and an estimate made of their likely consequence. The question being asked is: Are these flaws large enough to influence substantially the results obtained? The answer will depend on the nature of the problem. Occasional small and random errors in the data are unlikely to be important,

Table 14.2 Checklist for reviewing the study design

The research question
- Is the research question clearly stated?
- Has similar research been done before?
- How will the research add to current knowledge?
- Do the researchers have the necessary skills and expertise?
- Have appropriate collaborators been identified?

The data to be collected
- Is the set of data items clearly defined?
- Has the data set been checked against the study aims?
- Have potential sources of data been reviewed?
- Have the methods of measurement been described?
- Has the likely completeness of the data been assessed?
- Have validity and reliability been reviewed?
- Have off-the-shelf measures been investigated?

The research method
- Is the research method appropriate to the research question?
- Are all features of the method fully described?
- Have the members of the study group been adequately defined?
- Have potential pitfalls and sources of bias been reviewed?
- Has the need to generalise the findings been considered?
- Has a sample size calculation been carried out?
- Can enough subjects be recruited?
- Have the methods of stastistical analysis been considered?
- Has ethical permission been obtained?
- Has institutional approval been sought?

Practical design
- Has a protocol been developed?
- Has a realistic timetable been constructed?
- Have the resource implications been considered?
- Have the data processing methods been developed?
- Have staff been adequately trained?
- Have pilot studies been carried out?
- Is there a mechanism for reviewing progress?

whereas the selective loss of a particular type of patient, for example the more seriously ill or dead patients, could have a serious effect.

Be Prepared to Abandon a Project

Having come up with a good idea for a study, and when time and effort have been expended in developing it, the researcher may become particularly attached to it. However, some projects which initially look promising may turn out to be impossible, or to be so labour intensive that they are not worth completing. Research requires tenacity and perseverance, but also realism. If a major flaw in the design has emerged, or some vital items of data prove unavailable, then it is time to take stock. It may be that the project can be rescued through a modification of the design. But in some situations there is little for it than to recognise that a study will not work. Health professionals have limited opportunities for research and can thus ill afford to waste them on flawed research. It is far better to abandon at the design stage, than to discover halfway through data collection that the study is not feasible.

MONITOR THE CONDUCT OF THE STUDY

Even when they have been fully piloted, research studies inevitably encounter difficulties. To paraphrase Shakespeare: *'the course of true research never runs smooth'*. Problems should be expected and progress monitored regularly so that they can be detected. For example, in clinical trials patient recruitment often falls short of what was hoped. This would be easily identified if the numbers of patients recruited each month were recorded and compared with what had been predicted. In general, the study timetable needs to be inspected carefully, and all the key stages highlighted. These can be checked off as they occur, or action taken to ensure that problems encountered are tackled immediately.

Maintain Adequate Supervision

If you are carrying out all the stages of a research project by yourself, then you can deal with problems as they arise. But if one or more people are helping, then problems may have serious consequences. Sometimes an assistant will recognise a problem, deal with it when they can, and refer it to you if it is beyond their expertise. Unfortunately, such assistants are as rare as they are highly valued. More often the problem will be overlooked or ignored until it has festered away for some months. It may emerge when a major disaster occurs. Or worse, it may only be discovered during the analysis, when it is too late to do anything about it.

The only recourse is to ensure that staff are adequately trained, and are carefully supervised. Supervision does not mean checking up on mistakes, it means discussing study progress on a regular basis. The intention is to motivate and empower junior colleagues to respond to problems as they arise. People usually respond well to someone taking an interest in their work, particularly if the end result is to deal with a task with which they have been struggling.

Keep to the Original Plan

Once a project is underway changes should (almost) never be introduced to the design. New ideas may come to mind because of the attention given to a study in the early phases of data collection. These may suggest additional questions that can be asked, or indicate modifications which could be made to the study method. But changes made when a study is underway are likely to be poorly thought through and will not have been tested in a pilot study. In consequence, changes adopted in an attempt to improve a study may well end up ruining it. Far better to ensure that the design is fully thought through before the study is begun in earnest.

Changes are often proposed because difficulties are encountered either in obtaining data or in maintaining the required quality of the data. But these are the types of problem which should have been resolved in the pilot study. Introducing changes to the way data is collected could result in two different (and potentially incompatible) sets of data. If this occurs, either the two sets of data must be analysed and presented separately, or the first set must be discarded. To avoid the pain of having to throw data away, or confess that there were serious flaws in the design, there is no alternative but to test all features of the study in advance.

Keep a Study Log

During the course of a study, any problems occurring will need to be resolved. For example, if a patient moves house during a study, a decision will have to be made whether a journey to the new address is worthwhile. Or a doctor who had agreed to take part in a study may subsequently withdraw consent: should a substitute be sought? Whatever the decisions being made, it is good practice to record the reasons why actions were taken. Otherwise these will slip from the mind. Then when someone asks the key question: Why did we do it that way?, no one will remember the answer. There is little more certain in the conduct of a study than that the intimate details, which at the time were clear and self-evident, will be lost by the time it comes to writing the final report.

Finish

It may seem a little incongruous to talk about finishing a research project when it has just begun. The reason for emphasising it now is that *'it is too easy to dissipate energy in a multitude of unfinished and unpromising projects'* (7). Often the process of planning a project can suggest other interesting ideas for study. New ideas always seem more interesting, precisely because they are new. The enthusiasm for a study underway tends to be at a low ebb midway through data collection, making any new study doubly exciting. But if new ideas are followed up too quickly the first project may never be completed. Completion is much more than collecting the data: a study is not finished until it has been analysed, published and discussed by your colleagues (see Chapter 16). There are many filing cabinets filled with half planned and half completed studies. The only way to avoid adding to this litter of lost ideas is to stick with a study till it's done.

COMMENT

Developing the detailed design and monitoring the conduct of the study are crucial to the success of research. It is surprisingly easy to begin data collection before the design has been fully worked out. Often this is only discovered during data analysis, when it is too late to do anything about it. This can be prevented by an honest appraisal of the checklist given in Table 14.2. Monitoring of the study involves regular checks that the study is keeping up with the timetable which was drawn up. Unexpected problems often creep surreptitiously into a study, and can only be detected and corrected if the researcher is vigilant. Research, like all worthwhile endeavours, requires planning and application.

REFERENCES

1. Lowe, D. *Planning for Medical Research: A Practical Guide to Research Methods.* Middlesbrough: Astraglobe Limited, 1993: p iii.
2. Scottish Office. *Local Research Ethics Committees.* Edinburgh: HMSO, 1992.
3. Working Party of the BMA's Medical Ethics Committee. *Medical Ethics Today: Its Practice and Philosophy.* London: BMJ Publishing Group, 1993.
4. Garrett, TM, Baillie, HW and Garrett, RM. *Health Care Ethics: Principles and Problems* 2nd edn. Englewood Cliffs: Prentice-Hall, 1993.
5. Johnson, AG. *Pathways in Medical Ethics.* London: Edward Arnold, 1990.
6. The Data Protection Registrar. *The Data Protection Act 1984. Guideline No 1. An Introduction and Guide to the Act.* Wilmslow: Data Protection Registrar, 1985.
7. Calnan, J. *One Way To Do Research: The A–Z For Those Who Must.* London: William Heinemann Medical Books, 1976: p35.

Chapter 15

INTRODUCTION TO DATA ANALYSIS AND INTERPRETATION

The analysis and interpretation of data should be the most stimulating stage of a study: What have we found out? Does it challenge what was previously thought? Will it improve patient well-being? These are the types of questions which wait to be answered by the analysis. Data analysis need not be difficult to carry out, if it has been carefully planned. This chapter provides an introduction to the planning and conduct of the analysis of research studies. It does not describe the range of statistical methods which are available, as these would occupy a whole book. (Details of many good books on statistical methods are given in the Appendix at the end of this chapter.) Instead, this chapter describes essential ideas underlying statistical analysis, gives practical advice on how to conduct the analysis, and reviews how study findings can be interpreted.

ESSENTIAL IDEAS

Statistics resembles Tabasco sauce in its ability to produce a strong reaction in many people. Being listed at the end of the progression of lies and damned lies, statistics could be considered to have an image problem. This is unfortunate because statistical ideas and techniques have a vital role to play in research. Many of the ideas in statistical analysis have been developed to take account of the importance of the play of chance.

The Play of Chance

Chance affects all our lives. Unusual events do sometimes happen: someone will win the National Lottery, even though the chance of any one individual winning it is almost 14 million to one against. As well as the occurrence of unexpected events, the play of chance can mean that events which should have occurred sometimes do not. If you roll a six-sided die 10 times, you might expect to see at least one six. But there is a chance that no sixes will be seen.

These arguments about chance are all very well for gambling, but what do they have to do with research? The answer is that research is equally subject to the play of chance. Carrying out a survey, in which a sample of patients is selected, is analogous to drawing a hand of cards at bridge. In the game you would expect to get a mixture of cards including one or two kings and aces. You would also expect that in the next game the hand you are dealt will be quite different to the one you previously had (although again you would hope that it contained a few kings and aces). The hand that you get will broadly reflect the composition of the deck it came from, but its exact composition will be influenced by chance. Similarly, in a patient survey the group which is selected for the study should reflect the population from which it was obtained. But again, the exact composition will be influenced by chance. If a second sample were selected it would probably be broadly similar to the first, although it is likely to vary in many details. The problem then in interpreting the findings of a survey lies in deciding which results are truly meaningful, and which simply reflect the play of chance.

Chance does not only affect surveys, it applies with equal force to all research methods. The exact findings will be influenced by the play of chance, and repeated studies will often produce slightly different results. This is very clearly illustrated in the field of clinical trials where an individual treatment is sometimes investigated in several different studies. For example, a review of 33 separate studies of the effect of intravenous streptokinase for acute myocardial infarction found considerable variation between the individual trials (1). Some showed substantial benefit of treatment, others indicated a more modest effect, and a few suggested that the treatment might even be harmful. Taken together the studies show that treatment produces a moderate (25%) reduction in mortality. The results of individual studies are ranged about this overall result; most are close to it, but a few are some distance away. This variation between individual studies is exactly what would be expected by the play of chance. The importance of chance is that it can create interesting results where none exists, but it can also act to conceal important effects which do exist.

Probability: a Measure of Chance

Probability describes the chances of something happening. The chances of drawing the ace of spades from a deck of cards is $1/52$ (of the 52 cards which might be selected only one is the ace of spades). Probability is conventionally written as a decimal fraction: where 1/52 becomes 0.019. Probabilities can also be written as percentages, when 0.019 becomes 1.9%.

Probabilities can vary between zero (where an event will never happen) to 1.0 (where it is certain to happen). The Chinese emperor who wished to be remembered for his saying *'and this too shall pass away'* would have assigned a probability of 1.0 to the chances of his own empire passing away (and he would have been correct in doing so).

Interpreting probabilities is relatively straightforward. The probability that a man aged 30 will die over the next year is 0.001 (or equivalently 0.1%) (2). This only states what we already know, that young men are unlikely to die. In contrast, the probability that a man aged 80 will die in the next year is much higher at 0.12 (12%). This again shows what we know from experience, that as people get older their chances of dying increase. Indeed, by the age of 100 the probability that a man will die in the succeeding year is 0.41 (41%). In data analysis probabilities are interpreted in the same way: probabilities in the range 0.01 to 0.05 are considered to be small; and those in the range 0.2 to 0.5 are thought to be quite large.

Confidence Intervals

The influence of chance can make it difficult, simply by inspection, to decide what the findings from a study really mean. For example, a cohort study of patients with epilepsy showed a two-and-a-half-fold increase in the death rate (3). It is likely that if all the epileptics in Britain were followed up the overall result would differ from the risk observed in this study, although it is to be hoped not by very much. What can we say about what this overall value might be? Fortunately statistics provides a means of estimating a range within which we can be fairly certain this overall value might lie. The most commonly used range is the 95% confidence interval, which gives a range within which we can be 95% sure that the true value lies. The method of calculating the range is beyond the scope of the book, but is fully described in a book by Gardner and Altman (4). For the epilepsy patients mortality was increased by a factor of 2.5, and the 95% confidence interval was 2.1 to 2.9. Thus the increased mortality among all epileptics might be as low as twofold or nearly as high as threefold. Although we do not know exactly what the overall risk is, we are 95% sure it lies between a twofold and a threefold increase.

Confidence intervals can be obtained for all kinds of study results. They can be calculated for sample means, proportions, relative risks, and odds ratios. Although the details of the calculations differ, the interpretation of the range is always the same: the 95% confidence interval gives the range within which we can be 95% sure that the true value lies.

Hypothesis Testing

Many research studies ask questions like: *'Does fasting increase the frequency of accidental injury?'* (5) *'Are schizophrenic mothers more likely to have children with psychiatric disorders?'* (6) *'Are pregnant women who engage in strenuous physical activity more likely to have a spontaneous abortion?'* (7). These questions are of the form: Is this group different to that one? where the nature of the comparison group is implied in the question. The inclination might be to try to demonstrate that the two groups really do differ. Unfortunately, statistical methods cannot prove that two groups are different (indeed, research does not deal in proof). Instead, the best these methods can do is to show that it is extremely unlikely that the two groups are the same.

The approach then is first to propose that the two groups do not differ other than by chance. The next stage is to calculate how likely it is that the results could be due solely to the play of chance. This likelihood is expressed as a probability. The researcher usually does not believe that there is no difference, and may hope that the probability of the results being due to chance is small. Statistical methods provide the estimate of how likely it is that the two groups could differ in the way they do, assuming there was no real difference between them. (Technically the probability indicates how likely it is that results as extreme as those observed could be due to chance.) If the probability obtained is small, the decision is made that the two groups do differ.

The process of testing hypotheses can be illustrated with a study of whether a pressure-decreasing mattress could reduce the frequency of pressure sores in patients with femoral fractures (8). A randomised controlled clinical trial was conducted comparing the pressure-decreasing mattresses against those in current use. This found that only 25% of patients on the special mattresses had sores at one week, compared with 64% of patients on standard mattresses. Again, it is proposed that there was no difference between the two groups other than that occurring by chance. On this basis it was calculated that the probability was p=0.0043 of obtaining a difference as large as the one observed. The observed result is very unlikely to be due to chance (it would occur by chance less than one time in 200 fair trials). Thus it was concluded that the difference between the mattresses was real.

One unanswered question is how small does the probability (termed the p-value) have to be before chance is considered an unlikely explanation for the findings? By convention if p is less than 0.05 (written p<0.05) chance is rejected as a possible explanation. This rule is quite arbitrary, but it provides a convenient yardstick to assess p-values. The smaller the p-value, the less likely the results are to be due to chance. Thus when p<0.01 the results are considered highly significant and for p<0.001 very highly significant. In some publications the p-values are replaced by asterisks, with * meaning p<0.05 and *** corresponding to p<0.001. This practice has been described as being *'more appropriate to an hotel guide book than a serious scientific paper'* (9). It is much more informative to give the exact p-value.

Hypothesis tests have a wider use than just testing the differences between groups. They can be used to investigate questions like: Is the degree of compliance with therapy related to patients' beliefs about their illness? Does the length of time patients wait to be seen at a clinic affect their level of satisfaction with their treatment? These questions are concerned with whether two variables are related. They may involve the use of different statistical tests to those which compare groups, but the interpretation of the p-values is exactly the same.

P-values and Confidence Intervals

Testing hypotheses by calculating p-values and deriving confidence intervals might appear to be unrelated activities. But they are closely linked. This can be seen by considering the example of MMR (measles, mumps, rubella) vaccination in young children, where it is recommended that 90% should be immunised (10). Suppose that a survey of 100 children showed that only 80% had been vaccinated. Does this represent a true shortfall, or could it be due to the play of chance? The p-value approach would propose that there is no difference between the observed proportion and the stated target other than that due to chance. The statistical test would show a probability of p<0.05 that 80% of the children in the sample had been vaccinated if the overall value was 90%. This p-value is considered to be small, leading to the conclusion that there is a real shortfall in the rate of vaccination.

The confidence interval approach to these data would calculate the 95% confidence interval. It would range from 72% to 88%. This is the interval within which we are 95% sure that the true value will lie. But this range does not include the target of 90%, so we can conclude that 90% is unlikely to be the true value, i.e. that there is a real shortfall in rate of vaccination.

P-values and confidence intervals will always lead to similar conclusions, because of the underlying statistical theory (which we do not need to go into). Both will indicate whether the observed result could be due to chance. But confidence intervals have one advantage over p-values: they give the range in which the true value is likely to lie. It is because they give this extra information that confidence intervals are preferred to p-values by many medical journals.

PREPARING TO ANALYSE

Data analysis brings together statistical techniques and clinical experience: the statistics to show what is going on in the data, and the clinical experience to make sense of the statistical findings. This chapter does not review the statistical tests and graphical techniques which could be used in data analysis. These topics are well covered in the textbooks described in the Appendix. Instead, the following sections outline an approach to the analysis, giving practical advice on what should be done and how pitfalls can be avoided. These are topics which are sometimes less well covered in the available books, but are essential when conducting analyses. The researcher who does not feel confident about the analysis should think about contacting a statistician.

Choose a Statistical Package

The key to data analysis is a good statistical package. There are now several easy to use statistical packages for IBM compatible and Macintosh computers. It is far better to use a statistical package than some other package which can handle numerical data (e.g. databases or spreadsheets). These latter may offer some statistical facilities, but these will inevitably be limited, making it more difficult to carry out the analysis than with a dedicated statistical package.

Set up the Data File

The most time-consuming stage of data analysis is to get the data read correctly into the statistical package. Guidance on this is given in the manual which comes with the package. Basically the data items should be laid out in a fixed sequence with no items omitted. Most packages will read data if there is a space between each item. The computer knows which variable is which because of the sequence in which it reads the data. Gaps sometimes occur in the data because an item was not recorded for one of the study participants. However, a blank or missing item in the computer file can be catastrophic; it would lead to all the items after the gap being one place out. Missing items should be replaced with a missing values code (see Chapter 14). Once the sequence is correct there should be few problems.

Data files which contain more than eight or ten variables provide great scope for confusion. It can be difficult to identify which variable is which, and it is not unknown for the wrong variable to be analysed by mistake. This can be avoided by keeping a written record of the variables listed in sequence, together with a brief description of each. Many packages allow names to be given to variables, and adding these to the documentation can help to keep track of which variable is which. Sometimes related variables are given similar names. For example, when a patient's temperature is recorded six times during the day the variables might be named temp1, temp2, etc. At the time of naming there may have been a rationale for the terms used, but this will often be forgotten. Again, a written record will help identify variables if further analysis is conducted at a later date.

A First Look

No matter how carefully data have been collected and processed, there will inevitably be errors in the final data set. Some of these will be seen during analysis, because they represent impossible states: a diastolic blood pressure of 310 mm Hg; or a child aged 63 years. Thus before beginning the analysis it is worth having a quick look at each of the variables to check that they fall into the expected range. This can be achieved by plotting the data, say as a histogram or box-whisker plot, to see if there are any outlying values. These plots will also show whether the data take the range of values which would be expected. For example, diastolic blood pressure in men would be grouped around 80–85 mm Hg, with only a few having values as low as 60 or as high as 120 mm Hg.

Preliminary Recoding

Many variables, such as age and blood pressure, are distributed across a wide range, and almost everyone in the study will have a different value. It is often convenient in an analysis to group individuals into broad categories. For example, a survey of the frequency of chronic leg ulcers grouped individuals into five-year age bands (11). This clarified how rapidly the prevalence of disease increased with age.

To enable analyses of grouped data to be carried out, new variables need to be created, coding ranges to single values. Most statistical packages allow this to be carried out easily. Some of these packages allow the researcher to decide whether to replace the original data with the recoded values, or to create a new variable with the new data. It is advisable to create new variables; losing data is always a bad idea. Details of the new variables should be added to the listing of variables in the data file, otherwise the exact details of the coding will be lost in the recesses of memory.

DOING THE ANALYSIS

Data analysis begins with a review of the study aims, to identify what is needed to satisfy each aim. This will involve drawing up a set of tables and figures which need to be produced. Making progress on this before sitting down at the computer will save substantial amounts of time. The alternatives are either to gaze blankly at the screen or, much worse, to rush into complex statistical procedures. A cardinal rule of data analysis is keep it simple; only use sophisticated techniques when the data have been fully explored with simple ones.

Begin at the Beginning

All analyses should start by describing the number of patients (or other objects) in the study, summarising their basic characteristics: age, sex, disease groups, types of treatments. Initially these features should be looked at separately, and only after this should the relationship between variables be investigated: e.g. disease group by sex, treatment by disease group by age. The researcher is trying to get a feel for the data, for the main features of the study subjects. This makes it easier to interpret subsequent analyses.

Keep it Simple

Advances in computer technology have made it relatively easy to use complex statistical techniques. There is a temptation to start using them, in part because of the unspoken belief that the more sophisticated the technique the more convincing are the results it produces. This view is misplaced. Analysis should begin with the most simple methods of displaying the data, and move only gradually to more complicated techniques. Studies of the link between prenatal exposure to influenza and the development of schizophrenia provide one example of the dangers of using sophisticated techniques. An extensive review concluded that the research has *'generated a literature rich in complex statistical methods, inconsistencies, and contradictions . . . It has generated confusion'* (12). In general the more sophisticated the analysis, the easier it is to get it wrong.

Display Data

The amount of data collected in even a small study is so large that little can be gained just by looking at columns of numbers. Fortunately there are many graphical techniques which can be used to display the data. Graphs display data in a way which the mind can easily interpret. The use of graphs to represent data is one of the key stages in data analysis. As was said in a different context: *'a picture is worth a thousand words'*. Displaying data graphically allows the analyst to get a feel for the results. It will reveal relationships between variables and identify unusual or outlying observations. There is a wide range of graphical techniques which can be employed, described in books by Brown and Beck (13), Altman (14) and Bland (15).

Undertake the Analyses

Analysing data begins by displaying the data as graphs and summarising it in tables. The question then is which statistical tests should be used to identify the significant findings. Unfortunately, reviewing this topic is beyond the scope of this book; it would require a book to itself. For example, the book by Altman (14) describes the various types of data and the statistical tests most suited to each. But this book runs to some 600 pages. The only advice which can be given here on selecting statistical tests is to become familiar with the common tests by reading two or three of the textbooks listed at the end of the chapter. Picking the most appropriate test requires a familiarity with the tests so that judgement can be used. Because some statistical ideas are difficult to grasp, reading a single book will seldom be sufficient. In our experience it is helpful to read the explanations given in different textbooks, trying to fit them together.

Significance tests can readily be carried out using a statistical package. Current packages are designed to be easy to use. They come with manuals which explain how to apply each test, and many have an on-line help facility (you can ask the computer for advice on how to use the test). With the advent of *Windows*, doing the analysis only involves tiptoeing through the menu bars.

The ease with which sophisticated techniques can be used can create a problem: the tests can be used in inappropriate ways without the researcher being aware of this. All statistical tests make assumptions about the data being analysed. These need to be checked before tests are carried out. It is not advisable to use statistical tests unless you are thoroughly familiar with them, either by reading about them, or by discussing them with a statistician.

Annotate Printouts

Results of analyses can be displayed on the computer screen, or can be saved in a special file to be printed out later. Some statistical packages allow the researcher to select the analyses to be printed. Taking paper copies of the analyses saves writing them out by hand and keeps transcription errors to a minimum. However, as the analysis is extended, modified and repeated the amount of printout can grow into a confused heap of paper. Often it can be difficult even to decipher which variables were used in the analysis, far less decide what the purpose of it was. This can be avoided by labelling each analysis with the date and a brief description of what was done. Even better is to highlight the particular parts of the output that gave successful analyses, and to score out those parts where mistakes were made. (Experience shows that it is very easy to be a little confused at times during the analysis, and to produce output which makes no sense whatsoever.) The analyses can then be filed by date and by purpose so that the meaningful parts can easily be retrieved.

Watch the Missing Values Codes

Missing values are commonly coded 9 or 99 or 999 so that they are easily recognised. But they are sometimes overlooked when carrying out the analysis. Inadvertently including missing values codes as if they were actual values can wholly distort analyses. Most computer packages allow missing values to be specially marked so that they are omitted from analyses.

Missing data items cannot just be ignored. A few missing observations will be of little importance in a study of several hundred subjects. But if 20% or 30% of the observations for a variable are missing, analyses which are carried out could be flawed. The main concern is whether the subjects with missing data differ from those with complete information. Suppose that in a study of asthmatics, some peak flow readings could not be obtained because patients had died. Omitting these patients, who are likely to be the most seriously ill, could distort the study results. The extent of missing data should be reviewed to assess the extent to which it could influence the results.

Log the Findings

As the analysis proceeds and findings expected and unexpected emerge, it is worth recording in brief these findings. This can spark off new ideas for analysis, because the process of writing helps focus the mind on the results. Further, when the analysis becomes extensive, the notes present a convenient summary of what was found, and provide a logical trail through the analyses.

Avoid Data Torturing

When a time-consuming study has been completed the data are usually analysed with care to ensure that the findings are fully understood. For example, Jackson and colleagues (16) found that those who drink alcohol are on average at 40% lower risk of a heart attack than those who have never been drinkers. They naturally investigated what level of drinking was most protective and whether the effect was seen in both men and women (both sexes were found to be most protected by light to moderate drinking). This type of exploration of the exact nature of a finding is to be welcomed. But overenthusiastic analysis, in which every conceivable subgroup is explored in the hope that something will turn up, can be misleading: *study data, if manipulated in enough different ways, can be used to prove whatever the investigator wants to prove* (17). By investigating a sufficient number of subgroups, and even better leaving out some data points which don't fit the hypothesis, it will usually be possible to obtain a (spuriously) significant finding.

This caution against torturing does not mean that the data should not be fully explored nor that unexpected findings should be ignored. Quite the reverse. Data are always more interesting than could be imagined before they were obtained, and new insights will usually arise during analysis. But when a chance finding is made it should be recognised as such; an interesting observation which would need to be confirmed in a subsequent study. Exploratory analyses are sometimes described as fishing expeditions, and are an important part of research. They only come unstuck when the chance finding is presented as the very feature which is being sought: *'if the fishing expedition catches a boot, the fishermen should throw it back, not pretend they were fishing for boots'* (17).

Know When to Stop

When the analysis has explored each of the study aims and identified important findings about each, the analyst is faced with a problem: When do I stop? There are always further analyses that could be carried out, additional subgroups that could be investigated. Becoming lost in an analysis, particularly if the data set is large, is not just common: it is an occupational hazard. Even a comparatively modest study can lead to dozens of tables and graphs, keeping the researcher busy for days. The concern is not just with the time taken to produce these, but the longer time which their interpretation takes. To avoid being sucked into protracted data analysis, the researcher needs to ask at the start of a computer session: Why do I want to do this analysis? What will I get that is useful? If the answer is that it might completely change the interpretation of the study, then continue. But if it is only being done because it might be interesting, then it is probably time to stop. There will always be the opportunity to return to the analysis should mature reflection indicate this. Often the process of writing a paper or report will identify further limited analyses to be done. The important point is to stop the analysis and begin the writing to allow the opportunity for mature reflection.

INTERPRETING THE FINDINGS

In some instances deciding what a study has shown is straightforward. For example, a randomised controlled clinical trial gave powerful evidence that folic acid supplementation prevented neural tube defects (18). The study led immediately to the recommendation that all women planning a pregnancy should increase their intake of this vitamin (19). Unfortunately, such clear-cut results are rare. The interpretation of results needs time which is often not provided: *'it has always puzzled me that we are prepared to devote so much energy to obsessionally collecting the data, and yet spend so little time actually understanding it'* (20). Study findings need to be thought over at some length, their conclusions ruminated on. A number of separate activities need to be carried out:

- identify the serendipitous
- interpret with caution
- review statistical significance
- look for other explanations
- put the findings in context

Identify the Serendipitous

Data analysis usually throws up lots of findings, some interesting, others less so. The key findings should derive directly from the research questions which were defined at the start of the study. Whatever they are these findings need to be written out and mulled over, asking: Why did that happen? Why did it happen that way? What is the true importance of the result? Careful analysis will often reveal several surprises. But these fortuitous findings should have less weight attached to them than the results of analyses planned at the start of the study.

Interpret with Caution

Results need to be interpreted with caution, even when it appears clear what the findings mean. The sense of ownership, and even pride, which researchers have for their studies may lead to the findings being viewed too enthusiastically. Research is often carried out because the researcher has a pet theory and wishes to test whether or not it is true. There is a natural temptation to interpret research findings to support the theory. For example, a study was carried out to see whether newborn babies find their mother's nipple by smell (21). One breast, selected at random, was washed immediately after birth, the other being left untouched. Babies placed between the breasts showed a marked preference for the unwashed breast, leading the authors to conclude that the babies responded to differences in smell. This appears a likely explanation, but other explanations cannot be ruled out. Although the authors reported using an odourless soap, this does not exclude there being an aspect of smell or taste which deterred the babies from the washed breast. In addition to assessing the evidence, other explanations need to be sought.

Review Statistical Significance

Medical journals rightly place much emphasis on the statistical significance of study findings. However, it is possible to place too much reliance on statistical significance; it is only a tool and has limitations. These are:

- spurious significance
- importance not significance
- insufficient size
- borderline significance

Spurious Significance

Statistical significance gives some reassurance that a finding was not due to chance. But it does not guarantee this. Altman (22) describes a small study comparing the effects of two treatments on the frequency of male and female babies. One of the treatments gave the expected 50:50 ratio, but the other treatment yielded three times as many of the one sex as the other (the paper does not clarify which sex predominated). This difference was statistically significant ($p<0.05$). Being told that the study was carried out on cows not humans might lessen the reader's interest. But knowing that the treatment involved making the cows face north (group one) or south (group two) at the time of artificial insemination is a challenge to the reader's credulity. It is difficult to imagine how the direction of insemination could influence gender; it is much more likely that the result was a chance occurrence.

Spuriously significant results will inevitably be encountered from time to time. The reason for this lies in the nature of the p-value. The statement $p=0.05$ indicates that the observed result would occur by chance only one time in twenty. Suppose a study were carried out 20 times, say in different parts of the country. One study would be expected to give a significant result by chance alone. As there are many researchers actively conducting studies, there will be a fair number of spurious significances about. Smaller p-values, such as $p<0.01$ or $p<0.001$, provide more reassurance that the results are not due to chance. But even events which only happen one time in a thousand will occasionally occur.

Importance not Significance

The smaller the p-value the more confidence can be placed in a result. But this does not mean that the more significant a finding the more important it must be. If the sample size is large enough then even very weak effects can be highly statistically significant. For example, the annual mortality from breast cancer among women in England and Wales is 28.4 per 100 000, compared to 27.7 in Scotland (23). The difference between these rates is highly statistically significant (p<0.0001), but only because the rates are based on the observation of many millions of women. Practically speaking the rates are almost identical, especially in comparison with countries like Venezuela and Japan whose rates are less than 10 per 100 000. It is the size of an effect which determines its importance, not the level of significance.

Insufficient Size

Sometimes a study fails to find a significant effect when one had been expected. The absence of statistical significance does not necessarily mean that there was no effect, but rather that the study failed to detect one. This distinction is most clearly seen in clinical trials. A review was carried out of 71 studies which had failed to find a treatment effect (24). Most of these studies were too small to be able to detect clinically worthwhile effects; only 21 of the 71 would have detected a 50% improvement (e.g. a 50% reduction in mortality). The concern with sample size applies to all research methods. When negative findings are reported, the first question to be asked is whether the study was large enough to be able to show anything.

Borderline Significance

One difficulty which arises from the idea of significance is how to interpret a p-value which is just larger than 0.05. Intuitively there is little difference between a p-value of 0.049 and one of 0.051, yet the former would be declared statistically significant and the latter non-significant. P-values in the range 0.051 to 0.1 are described as being of borderline significance. Such a result provides a tantalising glimpse of a potentially important finding, although it could still be due to the play of chance. It is certainly possible that if the study had been larger, a significant result would have been obtained. To avoid tantalising borderline significance, studies should be planned with an eye to sample size.

Look for Other Explanations

Data interpretation should be undertaken with healthy scepticism. As one of the leading researchers of his day, Francis Crick, put it: *'misleading data, false ideas . . . occur in much if not all scientific work'* (25).

The importance of the play of chance was described above, but there are several possible explanations for the findings other than the direct interpretation, including:

- selection bias
- measurement bias
- regression to the mean
- association not causation
- trends over time
- confounding

Selection Bias

Patients who take part in studies often differ from those who do not. For example, a survey of the use of incontinence pads by women showed that those who were willing to be interviewed had much lower pad use than those who declined, especially in the age group 20–39 years (26). (This analysis was possible because incontinence pads are prescribed by doctors and data on them are routinely collected, enabling individual women to be identified.) This phenomenon is called selection bias.

Volunteering is a common cause of selection bias. It can even occur in research on children where the volunteering is done by the parents. One study of children taking part in a trial of asthma treatment showed that volunteering parents were *'significantly more socially disadvantaged and emotionally vulnerable'* than their non-volunteering counterparts (27).

A particularly important form of selection bias is the way it affects the types of patients seen in particular clinics. For example, one study investigated the patients being seen in 10 outpatient pain clinics. Although the clinics offered a similar range of services, there were substantial differences in the types of patients seen (28). This bias can lead to marked differences in the observed outcome at different clinics. Another study showed that specialist neonatal intensive care units had higher mortality rates than surrounding units. However, the specialist centres saw many more severely ill children which led to an increased death rate. When account was taken of this, by comparing children of similar severity, the specialist units were seen to do much better (29). The problem of case mix is a form of selection bias which is attracting increasing attention. It bedevils attempts to compare healthcare outcomes between clinicians, clinics and hospitals (30, 31).

Finally, it is worth noting that selection bias does not only operate on people, it can affect objects like casenotes. A study of the availability of casenotes found that: *'the retrieval of hospital notes was lower for deceased patients than for surviving patients'* (32). Whenever study results are being interpreted it is worth asking: What could have influenced the way these subjects were obtained? How might they differ from other groups with whom they are being compared?

Measurement Bias

Errors in the data are always a problem: some measurements will be made inaccurately, and questionnaires may be incorrectly filled in. If the information is being collected by interviewer then the way the questions are asked can influence the reply. Bias results when all, or most, of the errors are in the same direction. This could occur, for example, if a set of scales consistently overestimated weight. Or it could occur when participants' responses err in the same way. For example, people often understate the amount of alcohol they consume, and they may be economical with the truth on other sensitive matters such as how often they brush their teeth or the number of sexual partners they have had.

Measurement bias can be particularly important in studies in which two groups of subjects are being compared. Problems arise if the data are collected differently in the two groups. This can occur in quite subtle ways. Consider a study comparing women taking hormone replacement therapy (HRT) with a comparison group matched for age. Those on HRT are likely to be under regular medical supervision, so that minor illnesses and diseases at an early stage are more likely to be diagnosed. In consequence, HRT might appear associated with an increased burden of disease, even though this was in fact not the case.

Patient memory can also produce measurement bias, especially if those with a disease are compared to healthy controls. Those who are ill naturally seek an explanation for their disease, and will think through their recent history in some detail for possible causes. Therefore they will tend to remember and report details which healthy persons might forget.

In some circumstances blinding can be used to reduce measurement bias. If the interviewer is unaware which subjects are cases and which controls, then questions are more likely to be asked in the same way to both groups. Even with the best of intentions researchers can be biased in the way they collect data. These problems should be minimised at the stage of study design. The role of data interpretation is to assess the extent to which biases have crept in, and to determine the likely consequences.

The likelihood of measurement bias depends on the circumstances of measurement. When the data items are based on memory or opinion (e.g. clinical judgement), there is every chance that human frailty will be exposed. The more objective the measurement the less opportunity for error. But machines can be wrongly calibrated, or become faulty. It is best to assume that there is likely to be some bias, and devote energies to finding out how much. Occasional inaccuracies will usually be of little consequence. A few consistently high (or low) blood pressures in a study of several hundred persons is unlikely to be troublesome. There is no general rule to decide when bias is likely to be important. Instead, the researcher needs to review each finding and ask: Could this be substantially influenced by bias?

Regression to the Mean

Some variables can show large changes over time. For example, a blood pressure reading will depend on whether an individual feels stressed or has just run for a bus. When the blood pressure of a group of people is taken, some will have high values because of environmental influences; they will not be hypertensive. When these individuals are measured on a subsequent occasion many will have much lower readings because the external stressors will be absent. This tendency for some high values to revert to much lower ones is known as regression to the mean. It was first described more than 100 years ago when it was termed regression towards mediocrity (33). The phenomenon becomes important when comparisons are made between two successive measurements, such as before and after treatment for supposed hypertension. If those with high initial values are selected for treatment, then blood pressure will on average show a fall when measured a second time. This effect has been shown to occur in a number of studies of antihypertensive drugs, and has even been simulated with random numbers (34). Comparison of before and after measurements is a suspect procedure for any factor which can vary over time.

Association not Causation

Because two events are related does not mean that one causes the other. To illustrate this, Huff (35) discusses the question of whether body lice promote good health in the New Hebrides. It had been observed that those with good health had plenty of lice, whereas many sick persons had none. But before adding lice to the medical armamentarium, an alternative explanation needs to be considered. Infestation with lice was common at the time, so that most healthy people had them. However, it appeared that the body temperature of those with fever was unattractive to lice, and these patients were free of them. It was not that lice protect against disease, but that the absence of lice signals the presence of illness.

Trends over Time

Trends over time in the usage of health care facilities are notoriously difficult to interpret. For example, the 1970s and 1980s saw an epidemic of operations for glue ear (secretory otitis media). An examination of the evidence suggested that the prevalence of this condition had not increased. A number of separate factors were implicated including: *'the widespread introduction of audiometry; greater recognition . . . by general practitioners; the availability of more otolaryngologists; and technical advances such as the availability of . . . flanged tympanostomy tubes (grommets)'* (36). There was also the suggestion that surgeons needed to *'fill the vacuum caused by the decline in the number of adenotonsillectomies'*. The epidemic peaked in 1986 since when there has been a substantial fall in the number of operations, reflecting *'changes in clinical judgement by general practitioners and surgeons . . . and possibly of a reduced demand from parents'* (37).

The glue ear example may be a little unusual in the complex interplay of variables that influenced the frequency of operations. But it illustrates how more than one factor can change simultaneously. The example shows that usage of health care is not simply a question of patient need, but is affected by the attitudes of relatives, GPs, hospital clinicians and by technical developments. Trends over time have to be interpreted with great care.

Confounding

The association between two variables can sometimes be explained because both are related to a third variable. For example, one group of researchers found that general practitioners' work was related to the phases of the moon, being heaviest at the time of the full moon. The Transylvanian hypothesis, that human behaviour is influenced by the moon, was considered but finally rejected. Further analysis showed that *'any apparent effect could be explained by the occurrence of more bank holidays on the full moon days in our study period'* (38). This is an example of confounding.

Confounding can create effects where in reality none exist or can act to conceal relationships. Sometimes confounding is easy to spot. Leon (39) gives the example of the finding that people who carry matches are at an increased risk of lung cancer. It is more likely that the effect was due to smoking tobacco than to lighting matches.

Babies and Bathwater

The foregoing sections have pointed some of the many biases and flaws which can affect study findings. Researchers need to approach data interpretation with circumspection, alert to these pitfalls. But there is also the danger of overzealous criticism, of dismissing a study because of minor defects. Research studies are never perfect: response rates will fall short of 100%; some data items will be incorrectly recorded; opportunities for bias will be identified. The question is not whether a study is flawed; all studies are. What is important is whether the flaws are likely to be large enough to distort the findings. Thus rather than focusing on the existence of flaws, it is their magnitude which needs to be assessed. Findings are only discounted when there is reasonable suspicion that they are substantially affected by bias.

Put the Findings in Context

Identifying the main findings from the study is only one stage in data interpretation. They must be assessed to determine how they add to our understanding of health and health care and to identify the implications they have for service delivery. This is no simple task. Instead, it will involve reviewing each finding in turn, and asking questions like: What does this tell us that is new? What does it mean for health care delivery?

Findings can be compared with previous reports, asking whether the present study fits with what is already known. Results which confirm earlier studies are less likely to be due to chance than those which are totally unexpected. An isolated novel finding carries limited weight, whatever the probity of the study or the statistical significance of the findings. For example, a study was carried out into the practice of giving vitamin K to prevent haemolytic disease of the newborn (40). The finding that this was associated with an increased risk of cancer gave rise to considerable concern. But, because it was the first such report and because there was a lack of supporting evidence, a BMJ editorial concluded that: *'there are considerable doubts about whether the association is causal'* (41).

Findings are also interpreted in the light of established theory to determine the extent to which they could have been predicted. Those which meet with expectations will be more readily accepted than those which challenge the existing order. But this approach is double edged. Results may conflict with a theory, but it may not be immediately obvious whether it is the result or the theory which is at fault. Theories are often wrong, and studies which challenge them should be marked as *'controversial study, needs repetition'* rather than being abandoned.

In one field, that of assessing therapies, the rejection of evidence because of theory has been dubbed the tomato effect (42). The tomato is a member of the nightshade (*Solanacae*) family, many of whose members are poisonous or narcotic. The possibility that it might also be deadly led to the tomato being shunned in North America until the nineteenth century. This was despite its being widely consumed in Europe without ill effects. Indeed, the French even gave it the name *pomme d'amour* because of supposed aphrodisiac properties. In general, the findings from a study should not be ignored because they are in conflict with current wisdom. But neither should a single study, however positive, be taken as grounds for revolutionising the delivery of care. Better to adopt a cautious approach, integrating new results with existing evidence and theory.

COMMENT

Data analysis and interpretation, like medicine itself, is an art, albeit one which uses the concepts and techniques of science. Like many arts it requires knowledge and long practice to gain mastery. Conducting statistical tests to obtain a p-value is only a part of the task. Making sure that the analyses have been carried out correctly is probably more difficult than doing them. Equally difficult can be deciding what the findings really mean, and what implications they have for health care. Preparing these findings for publication is the subject of the next and final chapter.

APPENDIX: STATISTICAL TEXTBOOKS

This Appendix presents a list of statistics books. The list is far from complete, but it demonstrates the wealth of textbooks available. The books vary in the prior knowledge of statistics which they assume, and in the range of statistical tests which they describe. It is best to inspect several books to find those which best fit a researcher's needs. The list has been adapted from one published in *The Audit Handbook* (43), with permission.

Interpreting Data

How to Lie with Statistics, D Huff. London: Gollancz, 1954.
Humorous introduction to important statistical concepts and common pitfalls.
Facts from Figures, MJ Morony. London: Penguin, 1951.
Clear and interesting introduction to many statistical concepts, to methods of summarising and describing data, and to some statistical tests.
Making Sense of Data, JH Abramson. Oxford: Oxford University Press, 1988.
A self-instruction manual which asks the reader to interpret selected results. Many exercises are progressive as additional data shed new light on the initial findings. The reader is led gradually through more complex explanations. Highly recommended for those wishing to hone their skills in data interpretation.
Methodological Errors in Medical Research, B Andersen. Oxford: Blackwell, 1990.
Brief findings of published studies are described, and alternative explanations reviewed. Many dozens of studies are presented, covering the principal research methods and the common methodological pitfalls.

Simple Texts

Statistics without Tears, D Rowntree. London: Penguin, 1991.
Statistics at Square One, TDV Swinscow. London: BMJ, 1983.
Simple description of how to carry out basic statistical methods using a pocket calculator. Very little algebra is used, and clear explanations are given.
Statistics for the Terrified, G Kranzler and J Moursund. New Jersey: Prentice Hall, 1995.
Covers the basic statistical tests in plain language, with cartoons to lighten the text.
Medical Statistics on Microcomputers, RA Brown and J Swanson Beck. London: BMJ, 1990.
Clear description of approaches to data description and analysis. As the title implies, the book is designed for use with a statistical package on a microcomputer. This enables it to avoid formulae and to concentrate on the interpretation of findings.
Principles of Medical Statistics, AB Hill and ID Hill. London: Edward Arnold. 1991.
This is a revised edition of one of the most well known and widely used texts on medical statistics. It is easy to read and authoritative, covering all the standard statistical tests as well outlining the common pitfalls.

More Comprehensive Texts

These are slightly more advanced texts which use some algebra. They present methods of describing and summarising data, as well as a range of statistical tests.

An Introduction to Medical Statistics, M Bland. Oxford: Oxford University Press, 1995.

Medical Statistics: a Common-sense Approach, MJ Campbell and D Machin. Chichester: Wiley, 1990.
Practical Statistics for Medical Research, DG Altman. London: Chapman and Hall, 1991.
Statistics for Health Management and Research, M Woodward and LMA Francis. London: Arnold, 1988.
Interpretation and Uses of Medical Statistics, LE Daly, GJ Bourke and J McGilvary. Oxford: Blackwell, 1991.

Confidence Intervals

Statistics with Confidence, MJ Gardner and DG Altman. London: BMJ, 1990.
A review of methods of obtaining confidence intervals for a variety of summary statistics, e.g. mean, median, proportions and correlation coefficients.

More Advanced Texts

The following texts present some more specialised statistical methods. Despite being advanced they are clearly written to be understood by the non-mathematician.

Statistical Methods for Medical Investigations, BS Everitt. London: Arnold, 1989.
The Analysis of Contingency Tables, BS Everitt. London: Chapman & Hall, 1977.

Non-parametric Statistics

Non-parametric statistical tests are those which do not assume that the data follow a normal distribution or some other specified distribution (e.g. Poisson or binomial). These tests are ideally suited for data which are organised in rank order.

Nonparametric Statistics, S Seigel and NJ Catellan. New York: McGraw-Hill, 1988.
Introduction to Statistics: a Nonparametric Approach for the Social Sciences, C Leach. Chichester: Wiley, 1979.

REFERENCES

1. Lau, J, Antman, EM, Jimenez-Silva, J, Kupelnick, B, Mosteller, F and Chalmers, TC. Cumulative meta-analysis of therapeutic trials for myocardial infarction. *New England Journal of Medicine* 1992; **327**: 248–54.
2. Registrar General. *Life Tables: 1980–1982. First Supplement to the Hundred and Thirtythird Annual Report of the Registrar General for Scotland 1987*. Edinburgh: HMSO, 1987.
3. Cockerell, OC, Johnson, AL, Sander, JWAS, Hart, YM, Goodridge, DMG and Shorvon, SD. Mortality from epilepsy: results from a prospective population-based study. *Lancet* 1994; **344**: 918–21.

4. Gardner, MJ and Altman, DJ. *Statistics with Confidence*. London: British Medical Journal, 1990.
5. Langford, EJ, Ishaque, MA, Fothergill, J and Touquet, R. The effect of the fast of Ramadan on accident and emergency attendances. *Journal of the Royal Society of Medicine* 1994; **87**: 517–8.
6. Heston, LL. Psychiatric disorders in foster home reared children of schizophrenic mothers. *British Journal of Psychiatry* 1966; **112**: 819–25.
7. Eskenazi, B, Fenster, L, Wight, S, English, P, Windham, GC and Swan, SH. Physical exertion as a risk factor for spontaneous abortion. *Epidemiology* 1994; **5**: 6–13.
8. Hofman, A, Geelkerken, RH, Wille, J, Hamming, JJ, Hermans, J and Breslau, PJ. Pressure sores and pressure-decreasing mattresses: controlled clinical trial. *Lancet* 1994; **343**: 568–71.
9. Sprent, P. Some problems of statistical consultancy. *Journal of the Royal Statistical Society A* 1970; **133**: 139–48.
10. Department of Health, Welsh Office, Scottish Home and Health Department. *Immunisation Against Infectious Disease: 1990*. London: HMSO, 1990.
11. Nelzén, O, Bergqvist, D, Lindhagen, A and Hallböök, T. Chronic leg ulcers: an underestimated problem in primary health care among elderly patients. *Journal of Epidemiology and Community Health* 1991; **45**: 184–7.
12. Crow, TJ. Prenatal exposure to influenza as a cause of schizophrenia: there are inconsistencies and contradictions in the evidence. *British Journal of Psychiatry* 1994; **164**: 588–92.
13. Brown, RA, Swanson Beck, J. *Medical Statistics on Microcomputers*. London: British Medical Journal, 1990.
14. Altman, DG. *Practical Statistics for Medical Research*. London: Chapman and Hall, 1991.
15. Bland, N. *An Introduction to Medical Statistics* 2nd edn. Oxford: Oxford University Press, 1995.
16. Jackson, R, Scragg, R and Beaglehole, R. Alcohol consumption and risk of coronary heart disease. *British Medical Journal* 1991; **303**: 211–16.
17. Mills, JL. Data torturing. *New England Journal of Medicine* 1993; **329**: 1196–9.
18. MRC Vitamin Study Research Group. Prevention of neural tube defects: results of the Medical Research Council vitamin study. *Lancet* 1991; **338**: 131–7.
19. Wald, NJ and Bower, C. Folic acid and the prevention of neural tube defects. *British Medical Journal* 1995; **310**: 1019–20.
20. Persaud, R. Statistics: the glitter of the t table. *Lancet* 1993; **342**: 373.
21. Varendi, H, Porter, RH and Winberg, J. Does the newborn baby find the nipple by smell? *Lancet* 1994; **344**: 989–90.
22. Altman, DG. Statistics and ethics in medical research. VII Interpreting results. *British Medical Journal* 1980; **281**: 1612–14.
23. Cancer Research Campaign. Factsheet 6: breast cancer. In: *Facts on Cancer*. London: Cancer Research Campaign, 1991: 1–3.
24. Freiman, JA, Chalmers, TC, Smith, H Jr and Kuebler, RR. The importance of beta, the Type II error and sample size in the design and interpretation of the randomized control trial. Survey of 71 "negative" trials. *New England Journal of Medicine* 1978; **299**: 690–4.
25. Crick, F. *What Mad Pursuit*. London: Penguin, 1990: 67.
26. Sandvik, H and Hunskaar, S. Incontinence in women: different response

rates may introduce bias in community studies of pad consumption. *Journal of Epidemiology and Community Health* 1994; **48**: 419–22.

27. Harth, SC and Thong, YH. Sociodemographic and motivational characteristics of parents who volunteer their children for clinical research: a controlled study. *British Medical Journal* 1990; **300**: 1372–5.

28. Crombie, IK and Davies, HTO. Audit of outpatients: entering the loop. *British Medical Journal* 1991; **302**: 1437–9.

29. Pollack, MM, Alexander, SR, Clarke, N, Ruttimann, UE, Tesselaar, HM and Bachulis, AC. Improved outcomes from tertiary center pediatric intensive care: a statewide comparison of tertiary and nontertiary care facilities. *Critical Care Medicine* 1991; **19**: 150–9.

30. Bion, J. Outcomes in intensive care. *British Medical Journal* 1993; **307**: 953–4.

31. Orchard, C. Comparing healthcare outcomes. *British Medical Journal* 1994; **308**: 1493–6.

32. Gulliford, MC, Petruckevitch, A and Burney, PGJ. Hospital case notes and medical audit: evaluation of non-response. *British Medical Journal* 1991; **302**: 1128–9.

33. Bland, JM and Altman, DG. Regression towards the mean. *British Medical Journal* 1994; **308**: 1499.

34. Gill, JS, Zezulka, AV, Beevers, DG and Davies, P. Relation between initial blood pressure and its fall with treatment. *Lancet* 1985; **i**: 567–9.

35. Huff, D. *How to Lie with Statistics*. London: Gollancz, 1954: 98.

36. Black, N. Glue ear: the new dyslexia? *British Medical Journal* 1985; **290**: 1963–5.

37. Black, N. Surgery for glue ear: the English epidemic wanes. *Journal of Epidemiology and Community Health* 1995; **49**: 234–7.

38. Macdonald, L, Perkins, P, Pickering, R. Effect of the moon on general practitioners' on call work load. *Journal of Epidemiology and Community Health* 1994; **48**: 323–4.

39. Leon, DA. Failed or misleading adjustment for confounding. *Lancet* 1993; **342**: 479–81.

40. Golding, J, Greenwood, R, Birmingham, K and Mott, M. Childhood cancer, intramuscular vitamin K, and pethidine given during labour. *British Medical Journal* 1992; **305**: 341–6.

41. Draper, G and McNinch, A. Vitamin K for neonates: the controversy. *British Medical Journal* 1994; **308**: 867–8.

42. Goodwin, JS and Goodwin, JM. The tomato effect: rejection of highly efficacious therapies. *Journal of the American Medical Association* 1984; **251**: 2387–90.

43. Crombie, IK, Davies, HTO, Abraham, SCS and Florey, CdV. *The Audit Handbook: Improving Health Care through Clinical Audit*. Chichester: John Wiley & Sons, 1993.

Chapter 16

COMMUNICATING THE FINDINGS

Health services research is conducted with the aim of improving the delivery of health care. No matter how successful the research, improvements in care will only follow if the findings are communicated to health care professionals and managers. Publication should thus feature prominently in the research process. But, in comparison with the effort put into designing and conducting a study, relatively little time is spent on communicating its findings. The amount of interest in a research study falls steadily as the data are collected and the main analyses are conducted. Often, little enthusiasm is left to convert the results of the study into a form in which they can be conveyed to others.

The need to communicate does not imply that the researcher has to become some kind of scientific evangelist, promulgating findings from a soap-box. There are many well-established ways in which results can be disseminated: professional journals, conference lectures, conference posters, and reports to funding bodies. This chapter reviews how to prepare study findings for these channels of publication.

PREPARING TO PUBLISH

Whatever the form in which the findings of a study are to be published, some general guidance can be given:

- allow enough time
- answer four questions
- list the key findings
- prepare tables and graphs
- clarify the wider implications
- polish the first attempt

Allow Enough Time

Preparing the results of a study for publication takes time. Deciding what the study has shown and how best to convey the findings to others can be a challenging task. Constructing the tables and figures to illustrate these findings can be time consuming, as is the process of finding the correct words to describe the results. In consequence, allowance has to be made for this work when planning the study timetable. There is no generally accepted guidance for how much time should be set aside. But if a study has taken, say, 18 months to complete, from first conceiving the idea to plotting the last graph, then it seems wasteful not to spend another two or three months writing up the findings. Be generous when allowing for time to write up.

Answer Four Questions

Preparing a paper or lecture involves finding the answers to four questions (1):

- Why did you start?
- What did you do?
- What did you find out?
- What does it mean?

The questions follow the sequence in which the research should (ideally) be conducted. Arranging reports in this way makes it much easier for the reader or listener to understand what went on. Stating why it was done will set the study in context, and give a hint of what is to come. A description of how the study was carried out does much more than indicate the study methods, it indicates the types of data which will be presented. This makes it much easier to interpret the results when they are provided. Finally the results should be placed in the context of previous work to clarify the contribution made by the study.

List the Key Findings

The starting point for preparing a paper or a lecture is a list of the key findings. This is not a list of all the analyses which were performed. Instead, it comprises a concise statement of those few results which provide insights into health care. The process is one of reducing the mountain of computer printout to a short list of new and interesting findings. Then the tables and figures can be constructed to provide the results to support the key points.

The list of key findings is not intended to itemise everything that the study found. Instead, findings should be selected to form a logical development, the scientific equivalent of telling a story. Inevitably this will mean that some results will be omitted because they are not directly relevant to the theme(s) being developed. In short, do not try to cram everything into a single lecture or paper; doing so will usually confuse rather than inform an audience.

Prepare Tables and Graphs

Tables and graphs should be presented to illustrate the key findings. Different types of presentation (e.g. papers or lectures) will require different styles of tables and figures, but there are some common features. The information presented should allow the audience to draw their own conclusions about the study, without overwhelming them with data. Detailed results should be presented selectively. For example, in a survey of the frequency of urinary symptoms in men, age was thought to be an important factor, and several tables were subdivided by age (2). In contrast, a study of malnutrition among hospital patients was more concerned with the overall frequency of the condition and the actions taken to remedy it (3). Thus only one table was subdivided by age. In general, detailed results should only be presented when they support a key finding.

When presenting data in tables, it is important to check that the numbers add up. If there are 250 patients in the study, then the numbers of patients subdivided by age should add up to this total. Simple mistakes, caused for example by transcription errors, can call into question the validity of the whole study. A critical audience might wonder whether some patients were being left out, or added in, because this improved the results. Even a supportive audience will be left with doubts about the numeracy of the researcher and the amount of care taken in the analysis.

Clarify the Wider Implications

Having identified what appear to be the key findings, their importance needs to be elucidated. It is not enough to say: *'This is what I found'* and hope that the audience can work out its significance. The audience is more likely to dismiss the work as of little value. Instead, researchers should specify the consequences which arise from their findings, identifying the areas of health care for which they have relevance.

Polish the First Attempt

The most useful piece of advice when writing a paper or a lecture is to begin. What is written is much less important than that *something* has been written. The act of writing will help clarify your ideas, and it is much easier to see what improvements are needed when there is a draft copy to read. But having been produced, the first draft should be treated with suspicion, as something to be hacked about. It will almost certainly contain flaws in the logic and errors of fact, and it will abound with impenetrable English. Sections may be deleted or moved wholesale from one part of the paper to another. The final version will often look quite different, but it will only be achieved if the first has been drafted.

WRITING A PAPER

Writing the paper for the publication of your results is the culmination of a study. The task may appear daunting, but it can be broken down into a number of different activities.

Select the Journal

Medical journals vary substantially in the types of papers they publish. Some are highly specialised and like technical reports; others prefer studies of general clinical relevance. Thus the journal should be selected before the paper is written, to ensure the content is appropriate. It is worth spending some time in the library to identify possible journals and their preferences.

Journals also differ in the requirements they have for the structure of the manuscript: the length and layout of the text, the numbering of tables and graphs, and the format for references. These are usually given in guidelines which are published in the first issue of each year. The guidelines should be followed carefully to avoid antagonising the editor. One journal, the *British Medical Journal*, gives a particularly full set of instructions to authors, including checklists of criteria which are used in assessing the quality of the paper. Reading these will give a good indication of how papers should be written.

Write the Paper in Sections

Scientific papers have evolved a particular structure, comprising: title, abstract, introduction, methods, results, discussion, acknowledgements and references. They need not be written in the sequence given. Many researchers find it easier to start with the methods and results sections and then write the others. Whatever the order in which they are written, each of these sections must fulfil its set role.

Title

The title of a paper can attract or repulse potential readers. For example, Mayans and colleagues (4) could have used the lengthy and prosaic title: *'A randomised intervention trial on arthropod transmission of hepatitis B'*. Fortunately they used a snappier alternative: *'Do bedbugs transmit hepatitis B?'*, thereby increasing the number of people who will read their article. Short titles which indicate what the study is about will attract journal editors and readers.

Abstract

The abstract is by far the most important section of a paper. Other than the title, it is the only part that is read by most readers. If poorly written it will ensure the paper is not published. The abstract is *'a succinct precis of the paper'* (1), with one or two sentences covering each of the other sections. Many journals (such as the *British Medical Journal*) insist on a structured abstract, in which the sections of the paper are explicitly stated. Even if this is not the case, the abstract must convey the same information. This should be: the aim of the study, the research design, the setting and source of subjects, the measurements made, the results, and the conclusions and implications. The abstract should highlight the key findings and their implications, to make the reader want to enquire within.

Introduction

The introduction should be short, giving a brief background to the study and saying why it was carried out. It is not necessary to give an extensive review of the literature: additional references can be given in the discussion. Instead, the introduction should give sufficient information to show that there was a real need for the study. The background information should be selected and presented to make the reader think the research will be of value. This can be achieved by explaining why the topic is clinically important (e.g. in terms of mortality or morbidity from the condition) and how current knowledge suggests that there is an intriguing puzzle to be solved. In the introduction the author is making the case why anyone should bother to read the paper, and perhaps more importantly why it should be published. The introduction should end with a brief statement of the aims of the study.

Methods

Traditionally the methods section was intended to describe what was done in the study in sufficient detail so that others could replicate it if they wished. This is no longer the case; there is not enough space in modern journals for this amount of detail. Instead, enough information should be given to demonstrate that the study was conducted to a high standard. Some of the essential features are:

- the research design used
- the setting of the study (e.g. outpatient clinic, general practice)
- source, nature and number of the study subjects
- method of sampling
- the methods of obtaining data, including any questionnaires used
- the statistical methods used

Results

The results section begins with a broadbrush description of the study: the numbers of subjects and their principal features. Then it proceeds from the simple initial analyses to the more detailed and sophisticated ones. Only a limited amount of data can be presented, perhaps a maximum of six tables and figures, so these need to be selected with care. The aim is to lead your readers gradually into the data, presenting tables and graphs which lead them inexorably to the conclusions that you have already drawn. This is not always easy: *'to provide statistics is one thing: to induce people to believe in them is another'* (5). Explaining the logic behind the analyses and highlighting the key findings will help.

Discussion

The discussion fulfils several functions. It presents the main findings of the study but in summary form, avoiding repetition of results. Possible deficiencies in the methods used should be described, with an assessment of the size of effect (hopefully small) that these may have. Some authors are concerned that discussing deficiencies may somehow belittle their work. In practice the opposite is true: a frank discussion of (minor) defects gives a reader confidence in the researcher's honesty; the absence of reported defects raises suspicion.

The discussion should assess whether previous work is supported or contradicted by the results, and give an indication of the extent to which new ground has been broken. This gives authors the opportunity to emphasise the significance of their work. Sometimes a discussion concludes with suggestions for further research, although this can appear dull. It is too easy to conclude: *'therefore there is a need for further study'*. Better to finish with a bang than a whimper, and restate the important conclusion to which your work has led.

Expect Rejections

All researchers write some papers which are rejected by a journal as unsuitable. This does not mean that these papers contain no information of interest, or that they are fatally flawed. Most journals have many more papers submitted to them than they could publish and some, like the *British Medical Journal*, only have space for 10% of those received. Papers have more chance of being accepted if they are timely (i.e. deal with a topic that is currently of interest), are directly relevant to the principal readers of the journal, or have findings with important implications for clinical practice.

Many journals supply with the letter of rejection the comments of expert referees who have assessed the paper. These may indicate ways that the presentation and interpretation could be improved. Occasionally these comments show only that the referee completely failed to understand what was being said. The temptation to blame the referee for possessing fewer neurones than a snail should be resisted. If a reader has misunderstood, then the fault is probably in a lack of clarity or ambiguity of the text.

The rejection of a paper should be seen as a time for decision: What should I do next? One option is to appeal against the decision. This may be successful, particularly if you are certain that the referees' criticisms are misplaced. Appeals have to be tactfully phrased to avoid antagonising the editor. The alternative option is to ask a series of questions: Do I need to rewrite parts of it? Should different statistical methods be used?

Do the implications need emphasising? Which journal should I send it to next? If a research topic has been carefully selected and the study was well conducted, then it will almost certainly be published somewhere. It is a gratifying experience when a paper, which is published after previous rejection, attracts a lot of interest and becomes widely cited. Many researchers have had this experience.

PREPARING A LECTURE

A lecture to a conference or scientific meeting takes a quite different form to a paper submitted to a medical journal. A paper can be read at length, and its more difficult points pondered at leisure. In contrast, a lecture must be immediately comprehensible, and it must hold the listeners' attention. To be effective, a lecture must entertain. If the audience are bored they will hear only a fraction of what is said, and understand much less. Whether the talk contains vital new information or simply confirms what had previously been thought, a well crafted presentation will educate and stimulate the audience. Few of us are gifted orators, but attention to some key points can transform a hesitant and uninspiring lecture:

- prepare well
- provide an overview
- introduce the subject
- limit the data presented
- keep slides simple
- take care with overhead projectors
- do not read a manuscript
- annotate slides
- change pace
- have a take home message
- consider a handout
- rehearse

Prepare Well

A lecture which presents interesting material and runs to time has usually been crafted over many hours. The material has been carefully selected, the slides well drawn, and the talk rehearsed several times. This is particularly so when the speaker appears relaxed and makes a few off-the-cuff remarks. Often these remarks will have been carefully chosen and then rehearsed to capture the correct air of casualness. It is only when you wish to insult the audience that the slides can be hastily cobbled together with the hope that they will see you through the allotted time. Preparing a talk takes time; some speakers reckon that it takes one hour of preparation for each minute of presentation. This may be an overestimate, but it indicates the scale of effort required.

Provide an Overview

A colleague described the way he structured his lectures thus: *'First I tell them what I'm going to say, then I say it, and finally I tell them what I've told them.'* Providing a map of the lecture at the start, specifying the areas to be covered, can help the listener navigate the flow of information. It can prevent that dispiriting event, a bewildered audience wondering *'Why on earth have we moved onto this topic?'* The map is often arranged as a bullet list of areas to be covered. It can be repeated at points throughout the talk when passing from one major theme to the next.

Introduce the Subject

Some researchers are so deeply immersed in their subject that they assume that the background and aims of their research will also be well known to the audience. They tend to skip over these details, even though they are vital to the comprehension of the study findings. Instead, a brief introduction should be given, setting the scene for the lecture and indicating why the research was needed. Even if some in the audience are familiar with the topic, nothing is lost by bringing the information to the forefront of their minds.

Limit the Data Presented

Among the worst of lectures are those which are so filled with data, often presented at great speed, that they batter the audience into sub-mission. It is one of those ironies that the more information presented, the less will be remembered. There needs to be sufficient information to make a substantial talk, but only as much as can be presented clearly. It is better to finish one or two minutes early than to exceed the allotted time (everyone appreciates being released from the lecture hall a few minutes early). Thus the information to be presented should be pruned, removing items which are not essential to the main theme. As a general rule, about half the talk should be concerned with data, the balance being taken up with the introduction, an outline of the methods, and a discussion of the findings.

Keep Slides Simple

Tables with dozens of numbers and graphs with many different lines may be candidates for the *'most unreadable slide of the conference'* contest, but otherwise have little value. One easy way to irritate an audience is to show a slide containing a large amount of information, but ask them only to look at a single item. Why show all the others? Most tables should contain no more than three rows and three columns, and text slides should contain no more than about six lines. Text written in all capitals is difficult to read and should be avoided, even in titles. Graphs should be simple with clearly labelled axes, and if more than one curve is to be shown these should be drawn to be distinct.

Colour can add interest to a slide, but it has to be used with care. Some colours, such as blue, do not project well, making text and figures difficult to read. Too many colours, or changes in colours between slides, can be hard on the eyes. Better to pick two or three bright colours and use them consistently.

Take Care with Overhead Projectors

Using an overhead projector gives a touch of informality to a lecture. But this can go astray if the overheads are not neatly stored and placed deftly on the projector. Covering up part of the overhead and revealing it gradually can be irritating. Audiences don't like seeing a lecturer fiddling with transparencies, and tend to be impatient to see the concealed text. Handwritten overheads suggest that the talk may have been prepared at the last minute. These should be avoided, except for the occasional one presenting information which really is hot off the press. Another hazard of overhead projectors is for the speaker to obscure the slide by standing in front of the screen. Because the projectors sit on a desk at the front of the room, the lecturer needs to stand well to the side for the slides to be seen.

Do not Read a Manuscript

When preparing a lecture some researchers write in full what they intend to say, to ensure that all the points are covered and to guard against drying up. At its most extreme, some even read a prepared manuscript. This is a mistake. Written and spoken English are two quite different languages (6). Written English obeys rules of grammar. It consists of complete sentences which are punctuated to make sense to the eye, rather than to be easily spoken. In contrast, spoken English is seldom grammatical, and can use pauses and changes of speed and pitch to emphasise points. When a manuscript is read it sounds stilted, and is dull because it lacks the emphases which give speech life. Reading also makes it difficult to look directly at an audience. As with any other conversation, regular eye contact with your listeners helps keep their interest.

Annotate Slides

One way to avoid drying up is to make a paper copy of each slide and annotate it with the points to be made. This means that the lecturer has something to say to each slide, and there is no danger of forgetting any details. Further, because the points will be in note form, the lecturer will be encouraged to convert them into conventional spoken English. It can also be useful to omit one or two points from a text slide so that these can be mentioned while the audience is reading. This can give the impression that the speaker knows far more about the subject than is being presented.

Change Pace

The results of a study can often be presented as a series of tables, and many of these will have a similar layout. When shown, this repetition can be dull to the point of being soporific. A good lecture will have many changes of pace, in which tables are interspersed with text slides or graphs. Cartoons are a useful device for waking up an audience. These need only be vaguely relevant to the topic. The opportunity to laugh is usually sufficiently welcome that the audience will overlook the precise relevance of the joke. Another device is the pause. A few well-chosen pauses can generate a sense of anticipation so that listeners become eager to hear what comes next.

Have a Take Home Message

An acknowledged limitation of lectures is that those in the audience tend to miss some of the points made and to forget others. To ensure that they take something away it is worth emphasising a few key points at the end of the talk. Carefully phrased, these can leave the audience with the feeling: 'this researcher has made a contribution to the field'.

Consider a Handout

Some lecturers prepare a handout of key points and references to published work. These can be given out to participants who express interest at the end of a presentation. Handouts are more suited to small and informal lectures where there is easy contact with the audience. They may be less useful at large international gatherings, where formality may deter people from contacting a speaker.

Rehearse

Researchers tend not to be natural orators. But they can be good lecturers, if their material has been well prepared and the talk rehearsed. Rehearsal is not a matter of running through the slides and thinking, 'Yes, I know what I would say to these.' Rehearsal involves giving voice to these thoughts. It is remarkable how ideas which seemed clear in the mind become confused and uncertain when spoken aloud.

Rehearsals can take different forms. The researcher can speak to an empty room, just to check that the slides follow a logical sequence and last for approximately the correct time. Or the talk can be given to one or two close colleagues, who can comment on all aspects of the presentation. Finally, the lecture can be given to a local group, allowing the speaker to polish the delivery before giving it to some august national or international body.

PREPARING A POSTER

Posters are becoming more common and are being accorded a higher status than previously at many scientific meetings. They are no longer regarded as a consolation prize to those whose abstract was not selected for a lecture. Certainly, those attending the meeting who are interested in your poster have the opportunity to study it in detail and at their leisure, something denied them at conventional lectures. The poster is a different form of communication, but much of the guidance for lectures and papers applies: keep it simple; identify the key findings; follow the sequence of introduction, methods, results, discussion.

Planning the Layout

The size and shape of the poster will be set by the conference organisers. There is nothing wrong with using less space than has been allocated: this can make the poster more striking. But exceeding the stated dimensions could mean that the poster cannot be shown.

A common method of laying out a poster is to divide the material to be presented into six or eight blocks. A preliminary sketch on a large sheet of paper should help decide whether the overall display will be attractive. Some researchers organise their blocks in two rows to be read from left to right. Others prefer to arrange them as three or four columns to be read in sequence. As audiences seem to read posters in a somewhat haphazard way, glancing at tables or figures and skipping between introduction and conclusions, the actual choice of layout may matter less so long as there is an obvious logical structure. Because of the tendency of readers to flit about a poster, the panels needs to be largely self-explanatory.

Designing the Content

Posters, even more than lectures, need to have their content designed to be immediately interpretable. The title should be brief, but printed in large letters so that it can be easily read from 10 feet away. The key results should be presented as simple tables or graphs. Large blocks of text should not be used. These are unlikely to be read by even the most enthusiastic participant, and serve primarily to encourage the passers-by to keep on going. Instead, short statements can be made giving key points.

Posters provide the opportunity to display photographs, X-ray film, or copies of leaflets or short questionnaires. Carefully used these materials can be eye-catching. They can indicate the context of a study or the methods used more fully and concisely than text. Posters can also be enlivened by colour.

The main pitfall for posters is presenting too much information. More than the other forms of communication, posters need judicial selection of material. It is remarkable how little information is required to make a good poster. Thus when designing one, ask: Would the key finding stand out more if I cut out some of the detail? The answer is often 'yes', and some of the detail should be removed.

The acid test of a good poster is to display it for 30 seconds to a colleague who is unfamiliar with the work. If they can tell you what the study was about then the poster is successful. Listen to their description carefully, because the parts they omit or stumble over are likely to be the parts which need to be simplified.

REPORT TO THE FUNDING BODY

The organisations which give funding for research usually expect a report at the conclusion of the study. This report can be seen as a tedious waste of time because only one or two people will read it. Such a view could not be more misguided. Although only a few people will read it, they will do so with great care to ensure that their money has been spent wisely and to good effect. They will also remember the report and it will influence their decision should you seek funding from them at a later date.

The exact structure of the final report varies between funding bodies, and their individual requirements should be checked. Often the report need only be slightly longer than a published paper (about 2000 words), and may contain about six or eight tables and figures. Funding bodies seldom want comprehensive tomes of findings because, like other busy professionals, they do not have the time to read them. The advice given on how to write a paper will help in the preparation of these reports. However, the style of the report should recognise that the funding body's staff are not specialists in the field; some will be laypersons.

Whether or not the funding body requests one, it is a good idea to attach an executive summary. It is best to restrict this to a one-page document, laid out to be easily read. It focuses on the key findings, their implications, and the recommendations which follow from these.

COMMENT

Communicating research findings is a demanding task. It can often appear much more attractive to become involved in designing a new study than to labour on the report for a completed one. Yet this is essential if the research is not to suffer 'death by neglect' (7). Recognising the effort involved means that the researcher can plan the publication as part of the project.

The primary objective of health services research is to garner new knowledge which will improve the delivery of health care. The value of the research is the amount by which it improves care, which inevitably means changing current practice. Thus health services research does not only have to stand up to peer review and be published in scientific journals. The findings have to be sufficiently convincing, and must be presented with such clarity, to persuade professional colleagues to change the way they deliver care.

Writing papers and preparing lectures are skills which have to be learned through practice. But there are several books which give detailed advice on these tasks (8–12). Finally, those who wish to write clearly could do no better than read the revised version of Gowers' *The Complete Plain Words* (13).

REFERENCES

1. Anonymous. The reasons for writing. *British Medical Journal* 1965; **2**: 870.
2. Hunter, DJW, McKee, CM, Black, NA and Sanderson, CFB. Urinary symptoms: prevalence and severity in British men aged 55 and over. *Journal of Epidemiology and Community Health* 1994; **48**: 569–75.
3. McWhirter, JP and Pennington, CR. Incidence and recognition of malnutrition in hospital. *British Medical Journal* 1994; **308**: 945–8.
4. Mayans, MV, Hall, AJ, Inskip, HM, *et al.* Do bedbugs transmit hepatitis B? *Lancet* 1994; **343**: 761–3.
5. Calnan, J. *Coping with Research*. London: Heinemann, 1984: 37.
6. Calnan, J. *One Way To Do Research: The A–Z For Those Who Must*. London: William Heinemann Medical Books, 1976: 29.
7. Lock, S. Foreword. In: Hawkins, C and Sorgi, M, eds. *Research: How to Plan, Speak and Write about it*. Berlin: Springer-Verlag, 1985:
8. Hall, GM, ed. *How to Write a Paper*. London: British Medical Journal, 1994.
9. Hawkins, C and Sorgi, M, eds. *Research: How to Plan, Speak and Write about it*. Berlin: Springer-Verlag, 1985.
10. Day, RA. *How to Write and Publish a Scientific Paper* 3rd edn. Cambridge: Cambridge University Press, 1989.
11. Huth, EJ. *How to Write and Publish Papers in the Medical Sciences* 2nd edn. Baltimore: Williams & Wilkins, 1990.
12. Booth, V. *Communicating in Science: Writing a Scientific Paper and Speaking at Scientific Meetings* 2nd edn. Cambridge: Cambridge University Press, 1993.
13. Gowers, E. *The Complete Plain Words*. Revised by S Greenbaum and J Whitcup. London: Penguin, 1986.

INDEX

Index compiled by Caroline Sheard